THE PERSONAL
CARE ATTENDANT
GUIDE

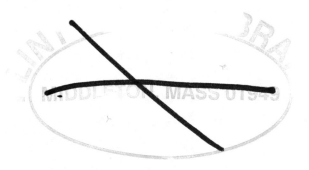

THE PERSONAL CARE ATTENDANT GUIDE

The Art of Finding, Keeping, or Being One

KATIE RODRIGUEZ BANISTER

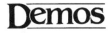

36214

Demos Medical Publishing
386 Park Avenue South, Suite 301
New York, NY 10016

Visit our website at www.demosmedpub.com

Library of Congress Cataloging-in-Publication Data
Banister, Katie Rodriguez.
  The personal care attendant guide : the art of finding, keeping, or being one / by Katie Rodriguez Banister.
    p. cm.
  Includes bibliographical references.
  ISBN-13: 978-1-932603-28-6 (pbk.)
  ISBN-10: 1-932603-28-X (pbk.)
  1. Home care services—Handbooks, manuals, etc. 2. Home health aides—Handbooks, manuals, etc. I. Title.
  RA645.3.B36 2006
  362.14—dc22

                                                                    2006020441

Special discounts on bulk quantities of Demos Medical Publishing books are available to corporations, professional associations, pharmaceutical companies, health care organizations, and other qualifying groups. For details, please contact:

Special Sales Department
Demos Medical Publishing
386 Park Avenue South, Suite 301
New York, NY 10016
Phone: 800-532-8663, 212-683-0072
Fax: 212-683-0118
Email: orderdept@demosmedpub.com

3 2126 00102 249 5

Made in the United States of America
06 07 08 09 10 5 4 3 2 1

About the Author

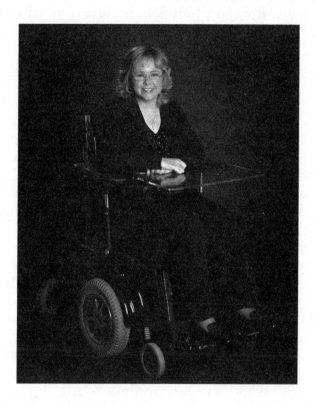

Katie Rodriguez Banister survived an auto accident in 1990 that left her a quadriplegic, paralyzed from the chest down. After 6 months of rehabilitation and 15 months residing with her parents, she returned to living independently in 1992.

Katie worked with the city of Webster Groves, Missouri for 5 years as their Access Coordinator. Prior to her accident, she was a latch-key director, a sales representative, a customer support representative, and social director.

Katie and her husband, Steve, co-founded Access-4-All, Inc., with a mission to educate and empower others through motivational speaking and disability education. Katie has authored *Aunt Katie's Visit*, an educational book for children, which has been enjoyed equally by parents, teachers, and librarians.

As a person who gives back to her community, Katie has been a member of the Recreation Council of the Greater St. Louis Board of Directors since 1992, where she has served two terms as president; and board member of Lifeskills in St. Louis. She was a board member and president of the Delta Center for Independent Living, and a board member of the VSA Arts of Missouri. Katie was also a performer and founding member of St. Louis' "DisAbility Project" and co-produced her own motivational video "Change Takes Time."

Katie has co-hosted the public access cable show "Beyond Barriers" and was on a 2003 commercial for the St. Louis Community College. Katie has been featured in local newspapers numerous times for her dedication to educating her community.

Katie's honors include a 2001 St. Louis Woman of Achievement; Missouri Jaycees 1998 Ten Outstanding Young Missourians; St. Louis Jaycees Jr. Chamber of Commerce 1995 Ten Outstanding Young St. Louisans; Missouri Governor's Council on Disability 1993 Advocate of the Year; Central Missouri State University Outstanding Freshman in the Department of Recreation 1983–84, and Kirkwood Missouri Jr. Miss 1982.

In addition to her responsibilities as president of Access-4-All, Inc., Katie is a dynamic speaker, author, consultant, and inventor of the Access-Sack. You can reach Katie at her website (www.access-4-all.com) or by e-mailing her at Katie@access-4-all.com.

Contents

Acknowledgments

There are many people I would like to thank for their loving input.

My family and especially my brother Tom, for without his help, my living independently would not have been possible.

Thank you to my dear friends Frank and Maxine Gilner for writing the Foreword to this book and for being true friends for almost 40 years now. The Rodriguez and Gilner families are one and the same. We have shared our Christmas trees and they have shared their matzo ball soup!

I am so grateful to my sister Eileen and her husband Bill for uprooting their lives to be by my side. Thank you to Monte and Phyllis Banister not only for producing Steve, the loving man I married, but for their financial help and loving enthusiasm about our work.

Thank you to Jan, my "Fairy God Mother" Hinkebein for helping me, whether she's driving me someplace, volunteering for so many of my projects, or doing whatever is asked of her.

I am grateful to my sister-in-law Susan Banister Ford for both helping me edit this book and for moving here from Florida, giving the St. Louis Banisters an opportunity to enjoy her husband Kimo and their four energetic children.

I wish to share my gratitude with the following people who have contributed to this book: Terri Venhaus, Rich Blakley, Rick Frame, Eric Westacott, Dick Hosty, Diane Riek, Ana and Steve Jennings, Bethany Geisler,

Tracy Fantini, Mike Sheller, Lisa Rustige, and Rhonda Dudley.

I wouldn't be the person I am today without the help of my therapist Susan. She knew me 3 months prior to my paralysis, and the journey has been a learning experience for both of us. Everybody needs someone to talk to honestly. It is through Susan that I know and love the person I am.

Thank you to my husband Steve, for loving my light and understanding my dark. I'm a better person because of him. He is patient, kind, and generous with his love. I'm enjoying this third dimension with him and look forward to what comes next.

This book is together because Tracy Fantini, Steve Banister, Sue Banister Ford, as well as John and Rose Saufnauer provided editorial assistance. Lance Tilford was a wonderful advisor as well.

This book is dedicated to the people who have come to my aid:

The Rodriguez family, the Banister family, Barnes-Jewish Hospital nursing staff, St. John's Mercy Medical Center's Department of Rehabilitation, especially Beth Crowner and Lori Burns. Dr. Bruce Bacon, Dr. Daniel Sohn, Dr. Ralph Clayman, Dr. Perry Lovinggood, Dr. Andrew Simonton, Dr. Dave Peterson, Dr. Karen Boesch, Dr. Mona Abouselman, Dr. Rodney Thorley, Dr. Susan Warshaw, Dr. Irini Veronikis, Dr. David Gray, Carla Walker, Jess Dashner, and all the of the Enabling Mobility Center staff, the staff at MediEquip, United Access staff, Joann Noll, and the fantastic women I've been assisted by, especially Amy La, Jennifer Payne, Refija Habibovic, Tracy Fantini, Melissa Bennett, Lisa Rustige, Rhonda Dudley, Cecelia Herbal, Chris Oliver, Emma Jones, Sue Whitton, Temia Keel, Kara, Suzanne Zimmerman, Sue Gomez, and Barb Patton. Also Sadye Gartland, Viky Abbott, Stacy Nard, Lisa "Woody" and Chris Ennis, Debbie Dubis Foster, Deb Bourbon and Pathways staff, and so many others!

Introduction

I wrote this book because . . . good help is hard to find. I should know. I have a spinal cord injury and am paralyzed from the chest down. I have been looking for help since 1992. But it hasn't been all bad. I have had many great personal care attendants and met some terrific people along the way.

Many people with and without disabilities, have asked me how I find my personal care attendants. This guide is my formal answer. It is my hope that the contents of this book will help people find the help they need. You may be a person with a disability needing an aide, or you may oversee the care of a loved one. Or, you may be a person who is considering working as a personal care attendant.

No "magic answers" make this intimate relationship work, but please allow me to share how I find my attendants. This is a personal guide on how to find and how to be a great personal care attendant.

This book contains:

- Personal advice on how to find a good attendant
- Suggestions and perspectives on how to be a good attendant
- Interviews with attendants and their perspectives
- Interviews with people with disabilities and their perspectives

- Helpful forms, including the Duty Spreadsheet, the Telephone Interview Sheet, an Employee Application, a Reference Information Sheet, a Police Authorization Background Check form and Additional Resources are found in the Appendix

It is important to me that both the person needing assistance and the person providing it realize the value of each other. An attendant is not meant to be a slave, and a person with a disability is not just a "person to take care of." Both individuals must respect each other. It is like a good marriage in the broadest sense. Both sides should really care for and try to understand the other's point of view.

Throughout this book, the terms personal care attendant (PCA), aide, caregiver, and attendant are used to describe those providing care for individuals who need it.

I don't have all the answers on how to find a great attendant or how to be one. What I do know is what I've learned from being a woman on wheels for more than 16 years now. I have also included some of my poetry throughout this guide.

So, please allow me to share how I find my personal care attendants with the hope that it may:

- Help you or a loved one live as independently as possible, or
- Help you become a great personal care attendant (PCA)

Foreword

We have known Katie Rodriguez Banister since she was 2 years old. She was a beautiful, bright, and happy child who grew into adulthood singing, dancing (so fast you couldn't always see her feet), and enjoying life.

She was always a very determined person, who set about doing things in an organized fashion . . . and got things done.

When she had her accident, we watched as she struggled to hold her own and deal with the news that she would not walk again. There were months of being strapped to machines, of surgeries, a halo attached to her head, and rehabilitation. Through it all, she focused on getting out of the hospital and building a life for herself.

Through the years of learning to cope as a quadriplegic, Katie grew in character and stature. She gives freely of her time to educate children how to relate to someone who has a disability. She serves the disabled community through Access-4-All. She continues to serve many not-for-profit boards and speaks to businesses and schools on diversity. Katie and her husband, Steve, have co-authored *Aunt Katie's Visit*, a children's book addressing the same theme. She has received numerous awards from the community for her efforts. You would like Katie. There is always an air of "can do" about her. It's uplifting to be in her presence.

This book brings Katie's intelligence, character, care for others, and "can do" spirit to a difficult and intimate problem of the severely physically and mentally challenged. It distills the years of trial-and-error, thoughtfulness, and sensitivity Katie experienced into a guide that provides practical advice for anyone seeking personal care from an attendant or desiring to provide that care.

The message of this book is clear: An able, respectful aide can diminish some of the worry and feelings of being overwhelmed by one's disability. This is made eminently clear in the personal statements of the aides and some of the people with disabilities included here. It is a step-by-step outline of what has to be done and how to do it. Katie's bottom line is always to find a way to live and enjoy life to the fullest!

Maxine W. Gilner, PhD
Frank H. Gilner, PhD, FAACP

CHAPTER 1

PREPARATION: ARE YOU READY TO HIRE A PERSONAL CARE ATTENDANT?

I miss the me
I used to be
Standing on my own.
But now wheels go round.
Freedom found.
Independence shown.

Issues to Consider When Hiring an Aide:
- Personal dependency
- Personal acceptance
- Time management
- Becoming an employer

Before you begin the process of hiring an agency or your own personal care attendant (PCA), several major issues must be considered. Living with a disability is scary. It can be frightening, because you don't always know who will walk through your door to assist you, whether it is a prospective aide applicant or a mystery aide from a home health agency. There is a good chance that many of us will face this type of dependency. For example, the Baby Boomers (those born following World War II, the generation from the late 1940s to the early 1960s) are quickly approaching the age at which assistance from others is going to be needed.

Asking for help and accepting it goes against our free will. It is human nature to want do things on your own. However, if you do need the help of others, you are not a weak person. So get that chip off your shoulder, if you have one, admit that you need help, and go on with the rest of your life. Do I like depending on others to help me every day with my most intimate needs? No, I don't! But not getting my bladder emptied or not taking a shower sound like pretty painful and stinky options!

People with disabilities are the largest minority group in the United States. When I became a member of this population in 1990, the estimated number was around 38 million. As I write, the current number is 58 million. The 1990 Americans with Disabilities Act recognizes two types of disabilities: physical and mental. But I see the breakdown as physical, sensory, cognitive, and emotional disabilities.

- *Physical Disabilities:*
  Physical disabilities affect a person's ability to move; they include:
  - Spinal cord injuries
  - Cerebral palsy
  - Spinal bifida
  - Muscular dystrophy
  - Bodily injuries
- *Sensory Impairments:*
  Sensory impairments affect a person's visual and auditory senses.

- *Cognitive Disabilities:*
  Cognitive disabilities affect a person's ability to mentally process information. These disabilities include:
  - Developmental and learning disabilities
  - Mild or severe mental retardation
- *Emotional Disabilities:*
  Emotional disabilities affect a person's ability to interact with others and society, such as:
  - Depression
  - Anxiety
  - Bipolar (manic-depressive) disorder

There is no such thing as an "easy" disability. They all force limitations on the people who have them, although some people who have an emotional disability can be more paralyzed than I am. My wheelchair and I can go anywhere I want to, provided the terrain is smooth. But I have heard of people with anxiety disorders who don't leave their home for days. (Appendix F, on page 131 of this guide, has a list of disability-related agencies and organizations that offer information and resources on some of these disabilities.)

Living with a disability requires two forms of acceptance. The first is the acceptance of who you are. I am now a person with a disability, but I am still basically the same person I was before I became disabled. However, my disability has educated me in so many wonderful ways. I've learned all about patience. I've also learned that life isn't always fair. Bad things happen everyday and to everyone. But the trick is to see the beauty in the bad and the value of all experiences. I've slowed down— well, my wheelchair made me slow down—and I now see the bonuses of my paralysis. A lot of good has come my way since becoming a "woman on wheels." (You can read more about my personal journey in Chapter Nine, This Wasn't What I Expected.)

Disabilities can happen to anyone, at any time, including those disabilities that occur at birth. There is an interesting debate on this very subject: People who are born with a disability have told me that they feel they may have it easier because they've never experienced life without a disability. On the other hand, I feel that being born with a disability would be harder because those folks have never experienced full abilities. Regardless of how you became a member of the disability culture, you are still a human being. If you incurred a disability, your body may not function the way it used to, but try to remember your inner being—your soul's essence can still be the same.

I must admit here that, even though I accept who I am, anger over loss is an issue I continually deal with and probably will for the rest of my life. But after 19 years of therapy and counseling, I have discovered that if I do not constructively deal with my anger, I pay a heavy price. I get headaches, I have stomach problems, my sleep suffers, and my ability to concentrate during the day is affected. Also my personal relationships with those I love suffer as well. So if you need help, ask for it or find it. Many self-help books, doctors, and counselors are out there to help you overcome difficult and stressful feelings. Get psychiatric help if you need to. I quickly learned that before I could fully invite others into my life to care for and help me, I had to know, understand, and accept who I am and my given circumstances. It is essential to deal with your anger and then put it aside in order to have healthy relationships with your personal care attendants.

The second form of acceptance is learning to accept the dependency upon others that you need to help you with your personal care needs. Prior to my paralysis, like most people, I was a fully independent person. I made a modest living, paid my bills, and had fun with my friends and family. Anyone who knew me before my paralysis will attest to the fact that I never sat still! I've always been fiercely independent and a woman on the go (probably going too fast). Paralysis not only showed me that I needed to slow down, but it taught me how to ask for help every day for the rest of my life. These two things are not easy to do, but I've learned how, and you will see how I do it throughout this guide. If I can do it, so can you. Have faith in yourself. You are more powerful than you think you are. Please remember and remind yourself that what you think creates your reality.

Something I discovered in my early days of independent living is that it's hard to function at full capacity in other areas of my life while looking for a personal care attendant. The process of looking for an aide is engaging and extremely time-consuming. I must allow myself adequate time to focus on this daunting task, and I can't commit to doing too much until I find someone to assist me. I have to balance finding an aide with the other activities of daily living. Balance is important. I can't be "on the go" while I'm looking for help because I have to stay home, answer phone calls from prospective aides, conduct interviews, check references, and train new hires.

My lifestyle is a part-time job, so when I'm looking for help, the rest of my life goes on hold. Susan, my therapist, helped me to acknowledge this issue. I deal with this aspect of independent living on a continuing basis. The alternative is living in a nursing home and, for me, that is a last resort. My independence is worth the time and effort it takes to maintain it.

Like it or not, as a person with a disability, you have become an employer. This will include all the duties that any employer undertakes—hiring, firing, scheduling, payroll, taxes, advertising, record keeping, and managing others.

A person cannot afford to have a casual approach to finding caregivers; you can't sit back and wait for an aide to magically appear. It's hard work. If you are the one who needs an attendant, you must be the person in charge of this process. Others can help you investigate options and possibilities, but you should have the final say, not family members or other care-givers. Be proactive. You might consider training your-self to be a good employer through reading books, tak-ing a human resource management class, or talking to other people with disabilities about how they manage their attendants.

If the person who needs a caregiver is unable to make decisions about his or her own care, the person with the utmost concern for the individual who needs personal care should be the one looking for the attendant.

My final words of advice on preparing yourself to bring personal care attendants into your life are: Be a person who others want to be around. This doesn't mean you have to always be "up" or "happy." If you are down one day, that's fine. We all have bad days. But snap your-self out of the "disability pity party." No one wants to hang out with someone who brings them down 24/7. If I'm sad, I cry, find someone who'll listen, and then I move on.

Crying is so important but it isn't easy for some people. I grew up hearing "Quit crying or I'll give you something to cry about." That was my father's way of coping with sad feel-ings. But those 19 years of therapy helped me to realize the value of a tear. Whenever I'm really mad and so angry that I want to ex-plode about everything, Susan would ask me, "Katie, have you been grieving?" My answer used to be "No" because grieving is hard work. Who wants to be sad? Society offers us all kinds of ways to avoid and mask our true feelings; substances like alcohol, tobacco, sugar, caffeine, and other drugs—prescription and nonprescription. But now I've learned to mourn my losses. Now, I cry with pride. But I still can't walk, and I'll always miss that ability. And that is something to cry about.

So, now having cried your eyes out, blown your nose, accepted your given situation and your dependency on others, you can now begin looking for a personal care attendant. I've made the process easy to follow with step-by-step instructions. You can do this. Really, you can. Read how I find my help, copy the easy-to-use forms in the back, and enjoy the stories from both caregivers and people who hire them. I use humor and my personal experiences in the hope that it will help you understand this interesting relationship and work environment.

When looking for your aide, remember this familiar saying: "Minds are like parachutes, they only function when open." Attendants come in all forms. There isn't an "attendant mold" out there. Caregivers must be helpful and dependable, but that aside, I've had attendants who were Asian, Muslim, African American, Jewish, Catholic, Mexican, Jehovah's Witness, Bosnian, married, single, athletic, conservative, independent, liberal, older, younger, simple, confused, shy, outgoing, co-dependent, messy, on-time, forgetful, nervous, insomniacs, exotic, petite, tacky, really tall, freckled, and people who were takers and many givers.

My point is, when looking for a caregiver, be open to all types of people. Let go of the prejudices and barriers that seem to set us apart from each other: religion, color, size, sexual orientation, political affiliations, and ethnicities. Life would be so boring if we were all alike. So— viva la difference!

All right, you are ready for the next step. Now go out there and find your attendant!

CHAPTER 2

FINDING A GOOD PERSONAL CARE ATTENDANT

My aide called, she can't come today.
She probably wants to go out and play.
Or maybe she's under and feeling quite sickly.
Yes, assumptions can be made too quickly.
But damn it! I also want to get out
So I sit inside and start to pout.
Other people can go out and explore.
They can open their own front door.
But I need someone to do that for me.
When no one comes, I'm so lonely.

There are two ways you can to find attendants: you can use attendant-providing agencies or hire your own attendant. Agencies are listed in the Yellow Pages under "Nursing" and "Home Health Services."

AGENCY-PROVIDED AIDES

Points to consider about using an agency to hire your aides are:

- They have a pool of prescreened workers to choose from
- They can usually provide back-up attendants on call
- They take care of the paperwork, insurance, taxes, and filing
- You can usually change attendants quickly
- The cost for an agency-provided aide averages $14 per hour (aides often make $7 to $10 an hour)
- A 4-hour minimum is often required for each visit

When considering an agency, don't be afraid to interview the agency. If they don't want to take time to answer your questions, it might not be an agency you want to use. Remember, we are talking about personal care. This is intimate work. You want to hire an agency that cares. Your first contact with an agency can often determine the kind of care you will get. If an agency gives you its full attention and answers your questions, I say go for it! Be firm and direct in asking these questions:

- How can you meet my needs?
- What advantages do you have over other agencies?
- How much is your staff paid, depending on their qualifications?
- What kind of training do you provide for your staff?
- Can I set my own schedule? (You should be able to)
- Can I meet the aide before he/she works for me?
- What if I do not like the person you send?
- Do you have back-up staff for emergencies or if someone calls in sick?
- What is the cost per hour?

- Do you have a minimum number of hours I have to pay for?
- Can someone work just a few hours for me?
- Do you offer health insurance to your employees?
- How are injuries on the job handled?
- Are you bonded and insured?
- Do you do background checks on your employees?

HIRING YOUR OWN AIDE

If you hire your own attendants:

- The aide will probably make more money working for you, rather than for an agency
- No hour minimums are required—you get what you want
- You or the aide must deal with taxes, Social Security, and other employment-related matters
- You may have to do all the training

PREPARING TO HIRE AN AIDE

To start, determine the needs of your body (see Section "Assessing Your Daily Needs" later in this chapter). Once you determine your physical needs, you can look for someone to meet them. When I first started out, I hired a full-time live-in attendant. That led to burnout on both sides after a few months. I then realized I had to find a different way to meet my needs. So I divided the work into three shifts: morning, afternoon, and overnight. I learned how to juggle a schedule of attendants who could do what needed to be done.

Scheduling is very important. For instance, I need my morning aide to be a morning person, or someone who is willing to adjust and get up early enough to be at my house by 7:30 a.m. I need my afternoon aide to be someone who likes to be on the go and has an adventurous aspect to his or her personality. My night aide must be a peaceful and easy-going person who can go to sleep, wake up, and help me with my personal care in the middle of the night and then go back to sleep.

You may have completely different scheduling. Figure out what works for you. There is no right way or wrong way. What's important is creating a way that is right for YOU.

COMPENSATION AND TAXES

Once you've decided what exactly you need in an aide, the next, and sometimes most difficult issue is that of compensation. For 10 years after my injury, I was on Medicaid and the state helped me pay for a morning attendant 5 days a week. This individual made about $6 per hour. I was also eligible for the state's Personal Care Assistant Program, administered by Paraquad, the local Center for Independent Living in St. Louis, Missouri. This gave me an afternoon attendant 6 hours a day, 5 days a week, who also made about $6 an hour. My family helped me cover the cost of my aide at night. My night aide started at $20 per night. After my lawsuit was settled in 1999, I formed a business and was able to compensate my attendants at a higher rate. When I couldn't pay my attendants a lot in the beginning, I treated them to gift certificates and small bonuses when I could. I also gave them a paid holiday when I could get a family member or friend to come in and help me on special occasions.

I've learned that most attendants are not in this business to make a lot of money. Yes, they need to be paid a fair wage for their services. But more often, they become attendants because they are caring individuals.

A fellow "quad" and I discussed the salary breakdown of attendant care and came up with the following table. These amounts are for the St. Louis area, and may vary state to state.

Going Rates for PCAs

We have found that if you pay	You will attract:
$20 an hour and up	Registered Nurses; people with medical experience and expertise
$12 to 16 an hour	Certified Nurses Assistants; people with extensive on-the-job experience
$7 to $10 an hour	People who may have little or no experience

Finally, reporting an attendant's income is a legal requirement. Taxes can be handled by the person hiring the aide or the aide who is doing the work. Consult with an accountant or use a payroll company to help you decide what is best for you and your situation.

I use a payroll company because juggling the paper work is not easy. It's one less headache. When I need help, I find it. You can too. Don't be intimidated. It can be accomplished using a slow and methodical process.

With the help of my accountant, I have included information on the tax forms that are used in the state of Missouri. Contact your local Department of Revenue to determine the tax responsibilities in your state.

Tax forms required on the federal level include:

- Form 1040 Schedule H—Household Employment Taxes
- Forms W-2, W-3, W-4

- Employment Eligibility Verification Form
- Form 940 Federal Unemployment
- Form 1099 Miscellaneous (for independent contractors)

Tax forms required by the state of Missouri and used as an example here include:

- Missouri Unemployment
- Missouri Withholding
- Form 2643 MO Tax Registration for Missouri Withholding

Some states may have city or county tax form requirements. Examples from St. Louis include:

- If you live in the City of St. Louis, the City of St. Louis requires employers to file Forms P-10 and W-10 quarterly, with an annual reconciliation report.
- If you live outside the City of St. Louis, but your employee is a resident of the City of St. Louis, the City of St. Louis requires Form W-10 to be filed quarterly, with an annual reconciliation report.

ASSESSING YOUR DAILY NEEDS

Before you can begin to look for attendant care, you must assess your daily needs. First, with a sense of total acceptance, I identify what must to be done by making a list of everything I need, starting from when I wake up to when I go to bed. I cover every detail from head to toe. My list includes:

- Bathing
- Dental care
- Hair care

- Beauty care
- Dressing
- Bladder and bowel care
- Transfers
- Range of motion and exercise
- Cooking and shopping
- Housekeeping, cleaning, laundry
- Transportation
- Work
- Recreation
- Paperwork (paying bills, record keeping, etc.)

Next, I create a Duty Spreadsheet showing the days of the week and each hour of the day (see Appendix A, on page 121).

Finally, I plug my list of needs into the time slots. This helps me to visualize what and when things need to be done. Once I arrange everything in order, I remind myself that the order can change from time to time. Being flexible allows you to handle changes, because change is life's only constant. With this in mind, I am prepared to enter the next phase in seeking assistance.

ADVERTISING: SENDING OUT MY SIGNAL

About a year before I became a quadriplegic, I was a sales representative for a leading business machine company. I lived in Columbia, Missouri, and my territory included fourteen southern Missouri counties. That job taught me what effective advertising and marketing was all about. Advertising of any kind must sound good, and it must be in the right place at the right time. When it comes to finding a good attendant, knowing what to say in an ad and placing the ad properly can make a difference.

I advertise with some information that is positive about me. Examples of words I use include "professional," "outgoing," "student," or "independent." Also, make use of humor. I frequently use "woman on wheels."

Or, I advertise with a positive word about the job, which could include "great location" or "flexible schedule."

Here are some examples:

- Aide for professional woman on wheels. Overnight 10 p.m. to 7 a.m. Some lifting and personal care. Reliable transportation needed.
- Aide for independent woman. Personal care, lifting, and driving. Noon to 6 p.m. Reliable transportation and dependable.

With every ad, of course, include your general location and a phone number where you can be reached by interested parties.

REMEMBER: A person with a disability is more than disabled, *and* a person with a disability can make for an interesting work opportunity!!!

PLACES TO ADVERTISE

Just like the old saying in real estate sales; the proper place for advertising depends on; Location, Location, Location! Where you advertise can affect your response.

- **City and County Newspapers:** While the average cost is high, it can be cost-effective to run an ad for 2 to 3 days—usually on Wednesday, Saturday, and Sunday. Remember to tell the person taking the ad that this is a position "in your home" and not for a business. This has saved me a few dollars.

I also recommend starting your ad with "Aide" or "Assistant" to ensure your ad will be listed first and be located alphabetically. Other lead words you can use include caregiver, therapeutic, part-/full-time position. You can also run ads in the "medical" section of the want ads. I've had good results from doing this. People who look for jobs in this section are more likely to have a medical or caregiving background. However, you may have to pay these people a higher wage because of their training and experience.

- **Community College and University Newspapers:** This type of advertising is usually low cost or sometimes free. Call the Employment Office at the school to run an ad in the campus newspaper. In addition, contact the Student Services Department for approval to post flyers at the Student Union and on other bulletin boards on campus. Students in allied health, occupational and physical therapy, massage and med tech studies are groups to target. However, although students can be great caregivers, their schedules change often and their availability can be very temporary, which makes it difficult to maintain consistency.

- **Church Bulletins:** Religious organizations often have bulletins or newsletters where attendants can be found by placing a small ad. I have often called local houses of worship to ask the staff if they might know of anyone who is looking for this type of work. This may be a free service, but ask to make sure.

- **Word-of-Mouth and E-mail:** This is often the best and least expensive way to find attendants because it doesn't cost a thing! If you need help, ask everyone—family, friends, local service agencies, business associates, doctors, and neighbors. You never know who you'll find when you ask "Do you know someone who can . . . ?"

THE PHONE INTERVIEW

On the day your ad appears in the paper, plan to be at home. When you need someone, and someone wants a job, answering the phone in person is much better than having an answering machine asking them to leave a message. To keep track of the people calling, I use a Telephone Interview Sheet (Appendix B, page 123) for each call. I keep copies by my phone with my writing brace close by. You could also enter this information in your computer and type as you talk.

The most important thing is consistency. Try to mention the same things in the same order to each caller so that you don't miss any part of your job description or forget to ask key questions. This is important for gathering the information you need when deciding whether or not to invite this person into your home for an interview.

Start the conversation with something like, "Let me tell you about me and what I'm looking for, and then you can tell me about you." With a statement like that, you are in control of the conversation, and it can also put the caller at ease.

Next, tell them your name, age, and the area in which you live. Then ask them where they live. If they live a great distance away from me, I usually end the interview, especially if I only need assistance for a few hours during the day. Additionally, I have learned that the closer they live, the easier it is for the attendant to be on time and work on a more permanent basis. The farther away, the easier it seems for some people to call at the last minute and tell you that they cannot report for duty.

However, if they live close-by, or they tell me that travel isn't a concern, then I continue the interview.

Next, discuss all of the tasks that need to be done:

- **Transfers:** First and foremost are your transfers in and out of your wheelchair. Ask "Can you lift, and are you strong?" I tell them my size and ability to assist by hanging on, letting them know that I need someone who knows how to do a lift using their legs and not their back. If you are a large person, make sure you mention the use of gait belts (used by an aide to help hold onto a client) or the use of a lift if it is needed.

- **Personal care:** Explain your bladder and bowel care. I have to be catheterized to empty my bladder every 5 hours. My attendant does so with a tube that is inserted into my urethra and drains into an attached bag. My bowel care consists of inserting a suppository inside my rectum, waiting 30 minutes, and then transferring me to my shower chair and letting nature take its course. After I describe my care, I ask them, "Would you be comfortable learning how to handle these intimate tasks?"

- **Duties:** Present a detailed account of your personal and household duties that need to be done, using the chart that you developed earlier. (See list on pages 14–15.) Mention everything you want the attendant to do. Honesty is definitely the best policy. Don't be afraid to share details here, especially if the applicant has experience or a medical background.

- **Driving:** If you need a driver, ask the caller if she would be comfortable driving

your vehicle (or, in my case, a big van),
Next, does she have a valid driver's
license? If you hire them, make a copy of
their license for your records. Also, be ab-
solutely sure to check with your insurance
company about having your aide drive
your vehicle. An additional cost may be
added to your policy premium, but you
want to make sure your vehicle is covered
no matter who drives it.

Most of the time, I hire people with their
own reliable transportation because I do
not live that close to a bus line. My attendants must be able to get to my house on
time and on their own. However, I did
hire a woman who was willing to walk a
distance and use public transportation,
and it worked successfully. It all depends
on the kind of public transportation available and where you live.

- **Time:** Describe your schedule and the required hours. Then ask the potential aide
  if she is available during those hours.

- **Money:** Inform the caller of the compensation you can offer and the method of payment. Some prospective attendants will
  want to work for "cash only." I avoid these
  candidates because typically, in my experience, they are on disability and/or receiv-
  ing public assistance or unemployment
  benefits. A good attendant will have a bank
  account in which she can deposit a check.
  My experience has also shown that people
  who want "cash only" are not as reliable
  as those who are paid by a company or
  personal check. Again, please make sure
  that you follow your state's tax laws regarding your employees and their com-

pensation. Work it out ahead of time as to who will be reporting an attendant's income. If there is an exchange of payment for services, the income must be reported, and taxes and Social Security payments must be considered.

Money management can be intimidating and confusing. Again, I recommend working through these issues with the help of a good accountant or payroll firm.

- **Ask and listen:** Ask the caller about her experiences working with people with disabilities. If someone doesn't have any experience, consider two things: I have found that people who have little or no experience with my condition can still make great attendants. But, if you have intensive medical needs, you may need someone with experience and specialized training.
  What the job really requires is a person with an open mind. Ask the applicant about their work experiences, current schedules, and current living arrangements. It is important to me to be up-front and honest with my information without scaring them into declining to accept the job. This is a fine line.
- **Smoking:** Cigarette smoking is a personal issue. I prefer attendants who do not smoke because I no longer smoke. I used to be a "social" smoker, and the last cigarette I had was the day of my accident. While I have had wonderful attendants who were smokers and didn't smoke

around me, finding cigarette butts in my
driveway often frustrated me.

- **Pets:** Some people have a very real fear of
animals. Potential attendants might have
allergies that could prevent them from
working in a home with pets. If you have
a pet, let your callers know.

If everything seems to be fine on the phone for both
of you, then you are ready to interview the candidate in
person. Fill out your Phone Interview Sheet, taking the
name, location, and phone number. Next:

- Agree on a day and time that would be
good for the both of you to meet.
- Give directions to meet you at your house
or some other convenient place, such as a
library or community center.
- Ask them to please call back if they have
to cancel or reschedule the interview.
- Ask them to bring along two work and
two personal references. This is so very
important! Don't forget to request this. It
demonstrates the accountability of the
prospective aide and maintains a professional relationship from your end.

Things to remember about the telephone interview:

- **A good phone interview can eliminate
wasted time.** You can get a general sense
of what the person is like through this
fairly lengthy discussion. People who don't
want to take the time to go through this
process won't make very good attendants.
- **If you feel "bad vibes" over the phone
from a potential attendant—and I have—
pay attention to these feelings.** Don't be
afraid or intimidated by these people. I

have had callers who were very controlling. They usually don't make it through
the phone interview.

- **Observe the callers' listening skills.** Are
they just talking about themselves, or are
they interested in you and what you are
looking for? I am not afraid to end a
phone interview if I'm not comfortable
with the caller. In a nice voice, I tell them,
"I don't think this will work out, but
thank you for calling" and end the call.
The person seeking the help must be the
one in charge of the conversation, the decision to set an interview date, and the
one to hire and fire an attendant. There
have been times I have had to simply
hang up the phone on some callers. Having Caller ID keeps me from having to
answer calls from pushy respondents who
try to call back.

- **You'll have some no-shows.** Many individuals who have passed my phone interview
did not arrive at the appointed time for an
interview or called to cancel their appointment. When this happens, their reasons
may vary, but it's still very rude. My time
is valuable, too! Sometimes I think people
enjoy talking with me on the phone, but
decide later that they don't want the work
and they feel bad about disappointing me.
So, be prepared. More than 80% of my interviews have been "no-shows." Don't get
discouraged. Pick up the phone, call someone else, and move on.

- **Keep track of those answering your ad
and who you hire.** I created a spreadsheet
on my computer and enter in any information I obtain. I do this because callers
whom I do not want to hire have called

back, months or years later, forgetting
they have talked to me already. Be prepared and find ways to protect yourself
from individuals who might attempt to
take advantage of you.

- **If you don't want to interview someone
  in your home, meet them at a restaurant,
  nearby library, community center, shopping mall, or other convenient public location.** You might need to have a two-step
  interview process. Do what makes you
  feel the safest. Your comfort and safety is
  the number-one priority.

THE FACE-TO-FACE INTERVIEW

There are four points to consider before your attendant
applicant arrives:

- **When.** Do you want to conduct the interview during the day or at night? I prefer
  interviewing during daylight hours, but
  this is not always possible, so I've learned
  to be flexible. Some people have other day
  jobs and can only meet at night.
- **Who.** Keep the interview relaxed, yet professional. Remember the person seeking
  assistance is the one who should be in
  control of the discussion. After all, you
  will sign the paychecks. I share my abilities with the applicant and review the duties of the position. During the discussion,
  we take turns communicating, but I lead
  the interview.
- **How.** Do you want to conduct the interview by yourself or with a friend or family member present in the home? This is
  an issue of safety and privacy. I wish I

could do everything on my own, but I can't. I also recognize that no matter how secure I feel on the inside, I'm vulnerable on the outside because of my paralysis. I like having another familiar person close at hand, just in case. I like my independence, but safety comes first. Once I invited a neighbor to come over to just hang around in the background while I interviewed an applicant.

- **Where.** Make your home inviting, clean, and tidy, with plenty of good lighting. Create a comfortable environment that someone will want to be a part of and work in. It doesn't have to be fancy, but it should be inviting.

When the applicant shows up for the interview, have her fill out:

- An Application Form (Appendix C, page 125)
- A Reference Form (Appendix D, page 127)
- A Police Record Check (Appendix E, page 129)

Sit comfortably while the applicant fills out your forms. I like to have my forms on a clipboard with a pen on my living room coffee table.

These are the questions I ask to make my hiring decisions. You may use these and edit them according to your circumstances.

- What experience do you have with people with disabilities?
- Why are you interested in being an aide?
- Are you looking for temporary or permanent work?
- What is your work and personal schedule?

- What do you do for fun?
- Describe how you manage time.
- In a way I am hiring your "hands" and must have things done a certain way. Can you take directions?
- How do you deal with constructive criticism?
- Are you a flexible person?
- How do you handle conflict?
- My family is important to me. Tell me about your family.
- What are your current living arrangements?
- What has been your greatest accomplishment?
- What are your strengths/weaknesses?
- Do you like to cook? When do you have your meals?
- If I am in a bad mood or stressed out and I ask you to do something differently from how you had been doing it, how would you react?
- On one hand, I will hire you and be your employer. On the other hand, there is a social aspect due to the intimacy of the job, with the possibility of a friendship. What are your thoughts on balancing the two?
- Are you a homebody or a person on the go?
- If you do an overnight shift for me, can you wake up in the middle of the night to help me and then go back to sleep?
- Tell me about a mistake you had at a previous job and how you handled it.
- Do you have any contagious or infectious diseases such as hepatitis, chronic mononucleosis, impetigo, etc.?

- Would a criminal background check be a problem for you?

Ask your questions and then simply listen. I pay close attention to body language. Do attendant applicants look you straight in the eye? Do they seem sincere in their responses? Are they relaxed and natural in responding to your questions? If they do all of the above, great! Or, do they blink their eyes or turn away when they answer a question? If they do this, that's not so great. Ten years of litigation and a few psychology courses have proven to me that if a person can't, or doesn't, look you in the eye, she might be hiding something.

I tell prospective attendants that I need an employee who will:

- Allow me to be me
- Respect my body
- Be a member of the household (i.e., a team player cooperating with my husband and other attendants)
- Be a person I can depend on
- Be able to plan ahead and commit to a given work schedule

It's important for me to have someone who listens to me, and again, who can look me straight in the eye. I need an aide who can communicate in a direct and positive way. I don't want someone who is negative and might bring me down. I'm dealing with enough already!

ASKING FOR REFERENCES

Okay, so you like the person. At the end of your interview, ask to see the two work and two personal references you asked her to bring. Have the applicant fill out the Reference Form (Appendix D, page 127). If she forgot to bring her reference information, it is a personal decision whether or not to give her another chance to provide the information. Can she look her references up in the phone book before she leaves? Can she go home and call you right back with the information?

I have given many of my attendant applicants a second chance. People can forget things. But I let them know that I must have their references in the next 24 hours in order to make my decision. If they are truly interested, they will do what has to be done and get you that information promptly.

It is very important to follow through and contact *all* references. I have done this by letter, phone, and e-mail. I recommend the telephone for time and convenience. When you call, ask the reference about the candidate's:

- Personality
- Dependability
- Reliability

Let the reference person know that the applicant will be assisting you in your home and that you have to know as much about this person as possible. If the applicant's reference is good, he or she will speak in a positive way at length about the applicant's abilities.

Many businesses cannot or will not give out any information beyond employment dates, due to potential legal ramifications. This is especially true of attendant-care agencies and nursing homes. An ideal reference is another employer with a disability or a client for whom the applicant has done private-duty work.

I cannot emphasize enough: One bad reference is one too many! I have given some attendants the benefit of the doubt and have always regretted it.

If the applicant has only one work or personal reference to offer, I would proceed with caution. Also be wary if the candidate only offers family members as references. If a prospective aide has no apparent employment history, he may be hiding something, unless he is a younger person with little or no work experience, or she has never had a job outside her home. These may be men, or more typically women, who have been homemakers. Don't write them off! Raising a family and running a household could make someone ready to be a caring and loyal attendant.

Finally, you may also want to run a police background check on the applicant. If so, have the applicant fill out and sign a release form (Appendix E, page 129).

THE TRAINING OF A NEW AIDE

I wish that every attendant could be psychic and know exactly what to do once he was hired. I'm sure some of them may be very intuitive, but they are not going to know exactly what your needs are. So—you have to tell them. You have to be specific with your instructions. You are the supervisor of your own care.

When you find a good candidate who you want to hire, he or she will have to "pass" a training period. Be prepared for a bumpy ride. Both of you may be eager to work together, but there is much to learn. You are exposing your body to someone new, and your aide must learn and complete so many new tasks.

I like to train on a one-on-one basis, where I am the instructor. But other training resources are available. Your local Center for Independent Living is an excellent resource. They often have personal care attendant programs. Check out our "Disability Resource List" (Appendix F, page 131) for other training suggestions.

All my new attendants start out the same way. First, I have the newly hired attendant come in and observe while a current attendant or my husband demonstrates how to transfer and catheterize me.

Then, I invite the attendant in training to transfer me in and out of my wheelchair to determine her comfort level. Sometimes, if I doubt their ability to lift me out of my wheelchair, I have them try to lift me during the first interview. This can save time for both of us because, if they are unable to do this, they are not going to be able to help me.

My method of transferring consists of my attendant putting my shins between her thighs to maintain control of my lower body. Then she points her feet in the direction in which she is going to transfer me. Next, I put my arm around her neck (giving them a hug) and put my chin on her shoulder to absorb the majority of my weight. My attendant stays bent over and uses her legs to bear the weight, instead of her back. We rock back and forth saying "1" . . . "2" . . . and move on "3."

I am very lucky that I am 4 foot and 11 inches tall, and have maintained a sensible weight since my accident in 1990. I also keep my arms in shape to maintain strength by using arm weights around my wrists, and I exercise most mornings. It isn't easy sitting full time. I watch what I eat and exercise every way I can. But like many women, I have a love/hate relationship with my physical being.

I have lost attendants who really wanted to work with me but could not do the transfer. If a person needing assistance is tall or of large size, he or she may battle this issue continuously. Transfer boards, gait belts, and Hoyer lifts may be helpful in meeting the transfer needs of people who need extra help getting out of their wheelchairs, and these devices may be purchased at local medical equipment suppliers.

The next step in training is the catheterization process, the way I empty my bladder. Again, I am "cathed" every 5 hours using a sterilized "cath kit." These types of kits can be purchased at medical supply businesses and often may be covered by Medicare. Paying out-of-pocket can be very expensive. Each cath kit contains gloves, antiseptic swabs, and a gelled catheter tube attached to a plastic bag. Everything is completely sterile. Using these cath kits has reduced the number of bladder infections I was plagued with before using them. I also take cranberry extract pills throughout the day to keep my bladder healthy.

The catheterization is then demonstrated while the attendant in training observes. I have lost potential attendants at this stage as well. There was one occasion when I really thought a candidate was going to pass out on me. After viewing the catheterization, she turned away saying, "I'm sorry. God I am so, so sorry!" and bolted out the door. It was too bad because she really wanted to work with me. But I think this type of work was just too intimate for her, although she had said she could do it. But saying so is often easier than seeing and doing.

If the prospective attendant can transfer me and handle the cath, I invite her to come back and *do* the cath with someone observing her. If all goes well, I have a new attendant! Yeah!!

Finally, have the new attendant fill out federal and state tax forms (see the section on Compensation and Taxes). Again, if necessary, you may want to consult with an accountant or consider using a payroll company to issue checks and deduct taxes. As a further incentive, I raise their pay after 90 days. This gives the aide something to look forward to and can save me a few bucks if the aide quits or is terminated before then.

> I have interviewed, hired, and trained several women who then didn't arrive for their first day of work! If they didn't want the job, all they would have had to do is say so. How hard is it to pick up a phone? This probably goes back to the "they didn't want to disappoint me" issue. Well, it's more disappointing when they don't show up or call, and it's just plain inconsiderate and rude! But what are you gonna do? People are people.

CAREGIVER TRAINING RECOMMENDATIONS

Take it easy and go slow. It is best to try not to plan a full schedule while looking for and training new attendants. Remind yourself that finding an attendant isn't an

easy process to work through, so try to cut yourself a little slack, and allow more time to do what must be done.

- **Be consistent.** Concentrate on your duty
  list and develop an effective schedule.
  Early on, I used a giant calendar on the
  wall with a dry-erase marker on a dan-
  gling string next to it so that everyone in
  the house was aware of what was happen-
  ing each day. Currently, I use a big desk-
  top organizer that I can write on. Try one
  of these methods or create your own way
  to get organized.
- **Learn to communicate well.** It is *vital* that
  you communicate your needs! Start off by
  doing things the right way from Day One.
  I try not to assume anything. My attendant is an extension of my being and is
  not there to just to "take care of me." Say
  what you want in a sincere way because
  no one likes to be yelled at or belittled.
- **Learn from each other.** Again: Say what
  you want, but also listen to your
  attendant. New attendants can bring in
  new ideas. I might like hearing about
  things of which I have little or no knowledge. We can all learn from each other, so
  keep an open mind.
- **Learn to manage conflict.** If you have a
  particular way of doing something, and an
  attendant feels it could be done another
  way, discuss this with him and work
  through it. But, if your aide neglects you
  and your requests, replace the attendant
  as soon as possible.
- **Control your situation.** The bottom line is
  you are in control of your body, your
  household, and how you want things

done. Again, welcome suggestions from your attendants. Many of my attendants have come to work with some great ideas. But when it comes down to it, you need certain things to be done certain ways. If you need to, remind your aide that your home is their work place.

- **Assess personality types.** If everyone had the same personality, the world would be a pretty boring and predictable place. There are two very general types of people, Type A (extroverts) and Type B (introverts). All of us are a combination and have characteristics of both types, but we may lean more toward one or the other.

  I am a Type A, for the most part. The majority of my attendants have been stronger B's but with some A in most of them. I have had a few attendants who were strong A's. This can be a difficult situation. As long as I have the final decision, I can get a lot accomplished with a Type A attendant.

  Type B personalities make wonderful attendants. They may move at a slower pace, but they are often people who are patient and adhere to a step-by-step routine process. They may be better listeners and be more nurturing.

  I also like to look at the applicant's birth date and consider aspects of their astrological signs. I know that everyone is unique. But access to this information gives me interesting insights. Astrology isn't for everyone, but I find it useful.

- **Keep time sheets.** To keep track of the number of hours your attendants work,

prepare a calendar for each shift each
month and put them on clipboards that
hang on a wall or that can be placed on a
table or counter in an undisturbed location. Each day my attendants sign in and
out. In this way, we both know what
hours have been worked. I use the calen-
dars to call in hours to the payroll company and retain them for a year in case of
any discrepancies.

Many combinations of traits and personalities make
people as diverse as they are. I have had to sift through
humanity to find the combinations that work for me and
my situation.

I believe I have talked to, interviewed, called references on, or hired over 400 women since my move to independent living. I have been very fortunate in securing
many wonderful women in my life to assist me. I prefer
women as attendants over men, and I have always liked
women doctors as well. This is a very personal choice. I
go with what's best for me. It's up to you to find what
works for you.

THINGS TO REMEMBER

- Attendants are an extension of your being.
  As people with disabilities, we must accept the fact that we need their assistance.
- Although you are physically dependent on
  a personal care attendant, he must create
  for you a feeling of safety, security, and
  serenity.
- A team player is the best kind of attendant.
- A wonderful friendship is always a bonus
  and a goal, but the attendant must be able
  to respect the personal boundaries of

those she is assisting. The work relationship must come first.

CONFRONTING ATTENDANTS

Your Body Is a Business

Confronting my attendants is probably the hardest part
of independent living for me. I make assumptions, and
it often back-fires on me. I give in again and again, and
I always regret it. Now, I've learned to stand-up for myself, so to speak (he-he).

If you need to correct or reprimand your attendant, do
it when you are on equal terms with her. You should be
seated upright so that you can talk eye-to-eye. Do not try
to discuss important issues when you are in the middle of
your more intimate care, such as bathing or during bowel
and bladder care. That is when you are more vulnerable.
The aide may feel he has power over you, and what you
have to discuss might not be taken seriously by him. Tell
your aide that you are willing to discuss their issues after
they are done with your care. Discuss important issues
when you are in a comfortable and empowering position.
For me, that is when I am fully dressed and upright in my
wheelchair and my personal care is complete.

You need care on a regular basis. Fully communicate
your needs from day one. Tell the aide that your body
needs certain care at certain times. If she does her duties,
she has a job. If not, you have to let her go. I have used
contracts in the past. Contracts are written agreements in
which the employer creates a list of job duties and the
compensation agreed on by both parties. I also recommend including the term "Duties as assigned," so that
you can ask your attendant to do the things you want
them to, providing its legal, moral and ethical. Both the
employer and employee agree to the conditions and sign
the document. If the aide refuses to sign the contract,
then it's time to find another aide!

Remember—You Are the Boss!

Some examples of situations I have had to confront include tardiness, asking for loans, lack of respect for my person and my opinions.

When an aide is late, I expect them to recognize their tardiness, say it won't happen again, and then be prompt the next time. I've had attendants who think arriving late is no big deal. So, after two or more late arrivals, I let them go. I'm not a charity case. I pay for what I need and that's the deal set during the interviewing process.

Attendants who ask to borrow money put me in an uncomfortable situation. I don't like doing it, and I almost always regret it. Because if they ask once, they're going to ask again. Attendants who have not paid me back are let go, and the funds are taken out of their final paycheck. I have learned to tell my attendants that I will not loan them money. Would a nursing home or home health agency give an employee a loan? I don't think so.

Some attendants don't respect my body. They forget to cover me after my shower or my personal care. I have little privacy when it comes to my body, so it is important that my aide show me respect in this regard. Learn to discuss these kinds of issues with your aide up front to avoid misunderstandings.

There have been times when my attendant has ignored me in public. One day while shopping, an attendant said to me, "Wait here, I have to go look for something," leaving me stranded, waiting for them. I said, "Excuse me, but I'm not paying you to do your shopping right now. I'm paying you to help me with mine." It's OK to be stern, but do so in a nice manner, showing respect for another human being. Don't insult your attendant, but don't let them walk all over you either.

Being chauffeured can be a challenging situation. My afternoon attendant drives my van and takes me to doctor's appointments, to speak at schools, and complete other errands as needed. Prior to my accident, I had driven a car for almost 10 years. Due to the damage of my left shoulder, I now choose to be a passenger. I have a lift on my van and a lock-down system for my wheelchair. After my aide secures my seatbelt, we take off.

Wherever I go, I have researched the location and have a travel route planned out. I don't like to waste time, and I know where I want to go. I have had attendants who don't listen to my directions and insist on going the way they want to. I have had to fire attendants who have this kind of attitude. Although I am open to discussing alternate driving routes, my aide should respect me, my vehicle, and how I want to reach my destinations.

Managing your own care is a daily challenge. In the next section, my friends on wheels share their perspectives.

PEOPLE WITH DISABILITIES SHARE THEIR PERSPECTIVE

I have met some really wonderful people since becoming a member of the disability culture in 1990. People like myself, who get frustrated with their limitations, yet life goes on. I asked them the following questions:

- How long have you used a personal care attendant?
- What are characteristics of a good aide?
- What type of people have been your attendants?
- What has your attendant done that shocked you?
- Who was your favorite attendant and why?
- Please share an interesting attendant experience.

Rich's Experiences

I have used personal care attendants for 24 years. Without them, I cannot work, attend school, get up in the morning, or go to bed at night. Without an attendant, I would be in a nursing home.

A good aide should be an individual who truly cares about your well-being and someone who doesn't provide services to you for the money alone. They do their job without complaining and direct supervision. They are honest and will not steal or lie. They don't complain about their personal problems while attending to my basic needs. Finally, above all, an aide should have a positive attitude.

My attendants have been black, white, and Asian. They've been fat and small, short and tall. I have fallen in love with them. They have fallen in love with me. They have been the most caring people in the world. Some have been really, really stupid. Many have been amazingly intelligent, yet did not have the self-confidence to fulfill their dreams. Some put my needs above their own. Others didn't have a clue what to do even after being trained! Although one gal stuffed cotton up her nose and made gagging noises during each bowel routine, she was excellent at her job and stayed with me for 2 years. Some got drunk every day. Some have been sweaty a lot and smelled just awful. One gave me encouragement to get out of bed when I was having my own personal time of self-pity.

I was so scared the time my aide became insanely drunk, grabbed my shotgun, loaded it, and accidentally discharged it in the house and didn't remember the incident the next day. One morning I really freaked out when I was in bed and my aide went into my living room and beat the hell out of his dog—there was nothing I could do to stop it. I dread the mornings my aide doesn't show up. No call, no warning. He just doesn't come, leaving me stranded in bed with the hope that someone will come to my rescue.

Who has been my favorite attendant? That would have to be my mom. Why? Because she was my mom!

Rick's Experiences

I have used a personal care attendant every day since I came home from the hospital after an accident four and a half years ago that left me a quadriplegic. My level of injury is at the third and fourth cervical vertebrae in my neck. I have learned that it's important for the Person with a Disability (PWD) to understand that an attendant is not a robot. Conversely, it's important for the attendant to understand (and accept) that it's not all about them. It's about the person they're assisting.

A good attendant situation is about compatibility and dependability. You're going to be spending a lot of time together, so compatibility is very important. The PWD is depending on you (that's why you're there), so an attendant must be dependable. It's a very sinking feeling when the clock strikes 8 a.m. and my attendant hasn't walked through the door and I'm left wondering if she's going to show up or not and if she doesn't, what am I going to do? It's also very important to the person you're assisting that he feels well taken care of.

A good relationship with your aide starts with an understanding of what needs to be done while remembering that one can't be overly demanding. Be sure to explain your needs clearly and in detail before hiring an attendant. Also, don't think that repeating something to make it clear is wrong. One of my frustrations is that, I explain to every attendant from the start that sometimes they will be here past their scheduled time to go home and that that time is not paid for. Despite this, when it does happen, every second or third week, I let them go early on another day to make up for it. Many of my attendants have stated during the interview that this arrangement would be fine, then three or four months later they start complaining about having to work past their scheduled leave time. Ugggggggh!

I've had attendants who were almost intuitive in knowing exactly what I wanted/needed and when I wanted/needed it. On the other hand, I've had attendants who had to be told what to do and when to do it every single day.

My favorite aide was my favorite because she was not only eager to do her job, but never complained. She pushed me to do what needed to be done even when I didn't feel like doing it.

I couldn't believe the time my aide ran up a $300 1-900-number telephone sex service bill! As far as the phone bill, I never paid it. We were able to explain to the phone company what happened, and they said if there are no more phone calls from my phone to those kinds of services that I don't have to worry about it. Whew!

Summers in Texas can be scorchers. My aide and I were running a little late one sunny morning in Dallas, but I knew my van had enough gas to get me to my appointment and that we would have to get gas for the trip back home. On the way back home, I asked my attendant how we were doing on gas, and she said she was waiting for a low gas indicator light to come on. I freaked out and said, "My van doesn't have one!" Then the van's engine began to sputter and turn off. My engineer's brain thought, "What next?" We were out of gas, and it was almost 100 degrees outside, which scared me because paralysis took away my ability to sweat. I get so sick when I'm overheated. We couldn't pull to the right because of a cement barrier, and we were two miles from an exit in either direction.

I asked my aid to try and start the van again. By the grace of God, it started and we were able to get to the next exit, but there wasn't a gas station in sight. Then I instructed my driver to turn right because it would put us in a downhill direction. We coasted downhill approximately one-half mile, caught a green light at an intersection at the bottom of the hill, and saw a gas station. It was certainly a miracle, and my attendant learned to keep a better eye on my van's gas tank.

Lastly, I have found that paying a monthly bonus in cash (if you can) works wonders. I tell all my attendants that, on top of their regular salary, I'll pay them a cash bonus every month based on their attendance and generally how good a job they're doing. This really has proven to be effective.

Terri's Experiences

In the past 14 years I've had attendants who were wonderful people, but it is such a shame that something so horrible (my spinal cord injury) had to happen for our paths to cross. My favorite attendant was my first, Michele. I instructed her how to do things my way, and she was extremely receptive. The hardest thing to do is to put your head in someone else's hands . . . . though it does help when an aide is great at hair styling!

An attendant should be reliable; when it's time to do a cath, she needs to be there. An attendant should be honest; while I'm waiting in one room for help, I have to hope that my aide isn't in another helping herself to anything that isn't hers.

On a funny note, I couldn't believe the time my aide told me that her family might be on Jerry Springer's show. It seems to me that the nicest people can come from the strangest families. Finally, it is because of my attendant that I can go to sleep at night, knowing she will be there in the morning. What more could you ask for?

Eric's Experiences

I am a quadriplegic and a practicing attorney who has been using attendants for 11 years. I've had attendants who were illiterate, incompetent, elderly, unreliable, or angry, and others who were dependable, understanding, hard-working, and even loving. I find these individuals mostly by word of mouth and recommendations from other disabled individuals. The best aide I ever had was great because he was dependable and reliable. I was so scared the time my aide did not show up and left me home alone in bed for an entire day without any way to contact anyone for help.

Dick's Experiences

I have cerebral palsy, which greatly affects my speech and ability to walk. I use attendants daily. If you want to help people like me, I have a few tips. One, knocking on my door before entering shows that you respect me and my space. Two, please ask me when I want to bathe, eat, sleep, or get up. I like to make my own decisions. As an advocate, I feel having full guardianship over someone doesn't mean you have full control over his personal life. I am my own person, and I need my personal space. Please respect me and my life.

Ana's and Steve's Experiences

My husband Steve has Friedreich's ataxia. This is a slowly progressive disorder of the nervous system and muscles. The disorder results in inability to coordinate voluntary muscle movements (ataxia). This condition is caused by degeneration of nerve tissue in the spinal cord and of nerves that extend to peripheral areas, such as the arms and legs. That ataxia affects upper and lower limbs, and the head and neck. There is also a particular loss of the sensations of touch and pressure in the arms and legs. Unlike some neurologic diseases, Friedreich's ataxia does not affect mental capacity.

Steve was diagnosed at the age of 14, and the lack of coordination became a problem when he turned 20. Steve's disability affects his speech and ability to push his manual wheelchair, but there's no stopping him from living a full life.

I acquired a spinal cord injury at the age of 18 and was independent until the age of 33, when I lost use of my left hand and broke my right arm. I need help getting bathed, dressed, cleaning around the house, and doing my laundry. Occasionally, my attendant picks up prescriptions or groceries for me.

The person who has helped me for the past few years is my favorite attendant. I can always count on her. If she is going to be late, she'll call to tell me, and she makes every effort to make up that time. She will change her schedule to come in earlier or stay later when I need her to do so. She willingly helps Steve when I am not physically able to do it. Steve's a pretty independent guy, but we all need help once in a while.

I have had my share of aides-from-hell, which makes me appreciate my current aide even more. I had an aide who came in and did nothing but sit at my kitchen table and do my new puzzle book. Soon after she started, I had to show her the door and tell her not to bother coming back. I called the attendant-care agency and told them not to send this woman to my home ever again. I need an aide who respects my belongings.

I had another aide who didn't show up or call, and then wondered why I didn't want her to come back to my home. The agency kept sending strangers to my home who broke my stuff, didn't say anything, and then stuck what they broke in a closet for me to find later. Needless to say, I changed agencies. I talked to the director of the agency I'm using now and made it clear to her that I don't want strangers coming in and out of my home. She agreed, and my current aide helps me both in the morning and at night. We keep a schedule that works for all of us.

IN CONCLUSION

My friends and I have been through a lot, and I'm sure our future attendant-care issues will be just as interesting— frustrating, but worth all the effort. I know that I want to live as independently as I can for as long as I can. And that includes having a good back-up plan of action.

CHAPTER 3

A GOOD BACK-UP PLAN

Keep this list of up-to-date information handy and let your caregivers know where you keep it. I like keeping this information in my wallet. Include the following:

- Your disability, condition and diagnosis
- A list of your medications
- Your medical, food and skin allergies
- Health conditions that might occur and what to do about them
- Emergency contact names and numbers of those closest to you
- Names of your doctor's hospitals and their telephone numbers
- Insurance information and related numbers or codes

When you have to let go of someone immediately, or when a regular attendant gets sick or cannot report for duty, having a person or two whom you can call upon in an emergency can keep your life rolling along. The best way to deal with this anxiety-producing situation is to prevent it.

It is highly unlikely that your current staff can be there 24/7. Emergencies happen. Schedules can change because of doctor appointments, child day-care problems, illness, funerals, and other uneasy times in our lives.

Finding a back-up aide isn't easy. Here are a few suggestions:

- Take time now to create a list of the most important tasks an attendant performs. Flexibility is important, because an emergency aide is often only available for a limited number of hours, and nonessential needs may not be met until you find a full-time aide.
- Develop a list of people who might be available for emergencies. People you could ask include family and friends; former attendants; people you go to school with, volunteer with, or know from church or social organizations; or other working attendants you know. When you ask if they are willing to help in an emergency situation, find out generally under what conditions or periods of time they would be available. Keep this information handy.
- Develop a short descriptive letter to recruit emergency back-up attendants to mail out to schools, resident apartment communities, the local Job Service office, grocery stores, and other places where you might place a quick ad.
- If the people you recruit for emergencies are people you don't know, take them

through your interviewing and training process. Keep their information and availability on your back-up list. You might want to hire them for full-time services in the future.

- Set aside some extra funding if you can to offer your back-ups a little extra for their time. Remember—if your schedule is disrupted, so is your back-up's.
- Update your emergency back-up list every 6 months or so. A brief phone call to see if your sources are still interested and available can save you a lot of frustration when you need someone on short notice. This is especially important because back-ups who are students have schedules that change every semester.

If you are reading this guide straight through, you have just gained an understanding of what you can do to find a personal care attendant. Next are suggestions and personal stories about being an attendant. You will find a great deal of humor throughout the next section. I find that humor is the best medicine.

CHAPTER 4

BEING A GOOD PERSONAL CARE ATTENDANT

The snow bound days remind me of
how vulnerable I've become.
Tons of snow
means I can't go,
I'm waiting for someone.
I watch the cars creep up the hill.
At least they're not sitting still
Like me who looks through a pane of glass
Waiting and hoping for time to pass.
Who will walk up my snowy ramp?
And enter in so cold and damp?
I'm sitting by the telephone
Expecting and wondering all alone.
I cannot do my personal care.
If no one shows I'm in despair.
I cannot get the things I need.
Does wanting help mean only greed?
The phone rings once, my speaker's on.
I say, "Hello" and the caller's gone.
It's scary when I have to wait.
It forces me to contemplate
Who will come and be relief?
Someone will, I have belief.

If you are contemplating becoming a personal care attendant, I applaud you! We need more people like you. As the Baby Boomers move into their retirement years, good help is going to be a necessity. It's important to most people I know to maintain as long, healthy, and independent a life as possible, for as long as possible. As a personal care attendant, you could be someone's key to independence!

ATTENDANT REQUIREMENTS

Right off the bat, I see three basic attendant requirements. Attendants should:

- Possess a genuine caring personality
- Be open to new experiences
- Be interested in more than just a job

Possess a Caring Personality

Although you are *caring for* someone, you are not there *to take care of them*. There is a difference. It's in how you perceive the person you're assisting. You take care of a baby or someone who is helpless. Chances are, if you currently are or want to be an aide, it will be with someone who is in charge of his or her own care, unless you are working for a family that is overseeing the care of a loved one. So please, care with sincerity and forget the pity!

Be Open to New Experiences

The only thing you can count on in life is change! And, that's an understatement when it comes to being a personal care attendant. Most working days are filled with bathing, dressing, chauffeuring, and keeping a household tidy. But in the business of caring for your fellow women or men, you have to be ready for anything.

Be Interested in More Than Just a Job

Being an attendant is different from working in a restaurant, a bank, or a department store, although the common thread running through all these jobs is customer service. What's unique about being an aide is that you are truly affecting someone's life. You can make a big difference every day!

IDEAL ATTENDANT CHARACTERISTICS

Attendants come in all shapes, sizes, ages, and color, with differing intellects, personalities, experiences, education, and levels of concern. The ideal personal care attendant should be:

- Dependable
- Honest
- Open
- Patient
- Flexible
- Truthful
- Sincere
- Positive
- Straightforward
- Nice
- Committed
- Steady
- Able to laugh
- Able to cry
- Faithful
- Organized
- Determined
- Uncomplaining

Anyone can have these traits. This isn't rocket science. If you want to be a caregiver, you have to give of yourself with a caring attitude. Anyone can be an attendant, if they have the right mindset and some formal or informal training.

Your mindset affects how you treat your clients. If you're always in a hurry, you don't finish your required tasks, and you see your job as a personal care attendant as a burden—QUIT! Seriously. This work isn't for you. At times, we all get frustrated with our jobs. That's human nature. But if you are an aide, of any kind, find a way to overcome the difficult duties in assisting your client or family member. No one likes dealing with bowel and bladder care, but it's often an essential part of the job. If you can't stand the steam during your client's shower, get out of the bathroom and find another place to work.

You really have to be a people person to be in this business. You have to have faith in others. You have to have hope for humanity. You have to care about yourself and your well being, as well as care for those you are assisting.

Some of my attendants and I have become great friends. The relationship starts out as employee and employer but, when you see the same person day after day for a year or more, good friendships can naturally happen. The best case is being friends while both individuals respect the working relationship.

Some of my aides have made me a part of their family, and they have become members of mine. While on duty, my aides have met my brothers and sister and my friends. On the flip side, my husband and I like to meet my attendants and take them and their family members out for a meal. This doesn't happen right away. It takes time for people to get to know each other.

ATTENDANT TRAINING

There are two types of training: formal and informal. About 5 or 6 years ago, I was approached by an instructor at one of our local community colleges who wanted to come up with a way to train students to be personal care attendants.

"Great," I thought. "This is gonna be awesome."

A committee was put together, a program was established, and students were interested. But who was going to pay for this attendant care training? The State couldn't. The students needing the training couldn't. Nursing agencies couldn't. People with disabilities couldn't either. So the program was shut down, and I was so disappointed.

Formal training is difficult to find. However, if you go to work for an agency or nursing home, they often do "on the job" training. As a new hire, you assist your clients with a "trainer" as a shadow, for a day or more. The Alzheimer's Association offers training on how to care for people with memory issues. Your local YMCA and Red Cross may provide classes on personal safety. Some Centers for Independent Living offer attendant care training as well. (See our Disability Resource List, Appendix F, page 131, for other contacts.)

I think informal training is best. This type of training is best obtained doing private-duty work, where the person needing the care or a family member trains you. If you can watch a routine and then do it safely and consistently, this work is for you. If you can handle messes and then clean them up, your abilities will be greatly appreciated. If you want to help a fellow human being live a better life, you can make a difference by reporting for duty each day you are committed to do so.

If my aide doesn't show up...

- My day is off to a bad start
- I'm stuck in bed until someone else can come in
- Other plans I had for the day are put on hold

Please remember, if you take on this responsibility, do so with the intention of showing up for work. Yes, things happen and circumstances change, but try to do your best in planning ahead so that someone who's waiting for you can depend on your arrival. However, if you can't make your next shift, call as soon as possible. Then different arrangements can be made so that your client's scheduled personal care is not disrupted. If you know the night before that your car isn't working or a family member is ill, please call your employer and let them know you may have difficulty being on time for your next shift, or coming in all together. This information is crucial to employer's personal care.

THE WRONG TYPES OF ATTENDANTS

Since 1992, I've had many good attendants who show up on time with a positive attitude and ready to assist me in whatever needs to be done. But I have also had attendants who were not so wonderful. These individuals fall into six attendant types I have categorized below. When I started summarizing the following attendant descriptions, I saw some of myself in a number of them and noticed that a few of my current attendants have some of these traits as well.

Listed below are extreme examples of attendant personalities and characteristics. I hope I don't offend anyone. But when I run across these types of attendants, they don't last more than two or three shifts due to the negative energy that surrounds them. These are examples on how *not* to be a personal-care attendant:

- **The Problem Queen/King.** This type of person calls at the last minute to say they can't come. They constantly complain, and they have a new ache or problem every day. Not a very happy person. This person has a problem, gets it taken care of, and then quickly finds another problem to complain about. They like the paycheck and are willing to work, but only on their terms.

- **The Slacker.** They are always 10 to 15 minutes late for their shift. They live in slow motion. Everything requires an incredible amount of time and effort. Putting away groceries can take an hour because they are always tired. They frequently complain and may try to claim more hours than they worked. This type of individual has used my address to hide from bill collectors by pretending to reside at my home, giving my address instead of their own.
- **The Controller.** These individuals think they know what's best. It's their way or no way, because they have more experience, education, or expertise than I, all of which they constantly remind me.
- **The Lucky Duck.** They let me know how lucky I am that they are there. They pretend that I require assistance only they can provide. They are interested in doing only the basics of my requirements, and don't see a positive future for me beyond my disability. They may take advantage by taking my things without asking such as food, clothing, make-up, office supplies, and the like.
- **The Dramatic Hero or Heroine.** These folks are self-righteous "do-gooders" and cannot easily admit fault. Their lives are one drama after another, and they are often the source of their own problems.
- **The Busybody.** They are overcommitted, and my care suffers. They want the hours and the pay, but won't take the time to fully complete the tasks that have to be

done. They are always in a hurry. This type of person could easily cause a bladder infection by rushing my cath, by placing the tube in the wrong place, and/or by not allowing my bladder enough time to fully empty.

- **The Moocher.** This personality doesn't show its face right away. It usually takes about 2 to 4 months to come out. Money is the problem. You give them a paycheck, but they always want more. Even if you can pay a good wage, it's never enough. If you have accumulated resources such as a nice house, jewelry, clothes, art, music, and other stuff, these folks often feel and project the attitude of, "If you have it, then you should give to me." They may want to be paid in cash or weekly, whereas most businesses I know pay by check every 2 weeks. The worst is when they ask to borrow money—and they always have heart breaking reasons why. They will often ask for a loan when you are in the middle of your shower or in some other vulnerable position and you are a "trapped" audience. These people can't manage their own money, and they want other people to solve their problems. They also take full advantage of elderly clients by "borrowing" (I call it stealing) their belongings, cash and/or using their client's credit card to buy personal things while shopping for their employer.

Sometimes, I feel as if I change my attendants as often as I change my underwear! People, schedules, and time all affect attendant-care candidates. This, in my opinion, is the most difficult factor in living with dependency on others. I have discovered that my day attendants usually last about 6 months to a year, and my overnight personnel are with me much longer, probably because the day job is more physically demanding. The night job takes someone who can go to sleep, wake up, do a cath, and then go back to sleep.

Certainly, not all my attendants have been attendants from hell. I have met some really fantastic and caring women over the years. Some have moved on, yet we still stay in contact through e-mail, holiday cards, or a phone call every once in a while.

> Remember, the relationship between a personal care attendant and the person he or she is assisting should be a give-and-take situation. Each can empower the other. Team work should be your mantra.

MY TRUE PERSONAL CARE ATTENDANT EXPERIENCES

To each of you present and future personal care attendants—

Make it attendant *care* not attendant *scare*!

These are a few of my true personal care attendant experiences. I have included them to inspire those of you learning to be a good personal care attendant. Most of the names have been changed to protect both parties.

While interviewing a potential attendant, she revealed that the last four clients she worked for had died, two of whom were not that old or sick. Because of that she had no references. Hmmmmm. I decided to pass on this candidate.

One day, my morning attendant Sharonna came in and gave me a shower, helped me with my bowel routine, and then took me to a luncheon. Our lunch consisted of a chicken and shrimp salad. Sharonna quickly put her shrimp on my plate, because she doesn't eat seafood. On the ride home, I said, "That salad was great." Sharonna with her quick wit said, "Yeah, well I guess I'll be seeing that again soon at your next shower!"

It was a cold and snowy night but Rhonda, my night attendant, managed to make her way to my house. As she took off her snowy shoes, I asked, "Is it pretty bad out there?" "Yes, it is," she answered. I said, "Thanks for coming. You really care about your job." "Well," Rhonda said with a smile. "You need me and frankly, I think the snow is rather pretty." Rhonda transferred me into my bed, cathed me, and we both went to sleep.

It takes a unique person to be an overnight attendant; she has to be able to go to sleep, wake up and cath me, and go back to sleep. Rhonda could do that with ease but I have had others who could not. My first overnight attendant would yell at me in the middle of the night saying, "Don't you know I have to go to work in the morning?" She had three jobs and was really overcommitted, and I had to let her go because I couldn't handle the guilt when I needed to pee!

I have had very "controlling" attendants who were usually older women and acted like mothers to me. This can be both good and bad. I love the general caring attitude and the desire to want to help. But it often comes with a price—the attitude of "I know what's best for you." Well, I have a mother and frankly, one's enough. Would you want two?

While sitting outside with my newly hired attendant, Sara, a bird flew over the two of us and pooped right on Sara's head! I tried not to laugh, but it was kind of funny. The next day Sara and I were again sitting outside and again a bird did the same thing to her. I'm not sure if it was the same bird, but Sara was pretty mad. About a week later, Sara left me, which turned out to be a good thing. Maybe the birds knew something I didn't!

Roxy came in to give me a shower. My routine consists of wetting my body down, turning off the water, shampooing my hair, soaping up my body, then turning the water on and rinsing me clean. Roxy wet my body down, but left the water running while she did the rest. By the time it came to the rinsing part, the water was ice cold! Believe me when I say, I was awake after that shower! Roxy never let the water run on again.

One day, I noticed that I had money missing from my wallet. In order to be fair to everyone, I decided to file a police report. My staff of four agreed to go to the police station to be questioned, but my relationship with one in particular changed drastically. Cheryl could no longer look me in the eye. After the police interviews were complete, a police officer called me and said, "Katie, we feel that all the women had access to your wallet at one time or another. I might suggest purchasing a lock box." I really liked that idea and use it to this day. I asked the officer, "Who do you think stole my money?" and he replied "Well, I think it was Cheryl." "OK, thank you." Not 5 minutes later the phone rang. "Hello?" "Hi, it's Cheryl. Look, I need to move on. My mom needs my help around the house, so I hope you can find someone to replace me. Bye." And she hung up. Most of my bad attendants have fired themselves.

I have had three very different traveling experiences with attendants. My first trip was to Disney World and to enjoy Steve's sister Sue's wedding celebration in Florida. I had never been to Disney World before and was very excited about going. Lisa (my aide) and Steve got along wonderfully. We spent 4 days touring the grounds. Each morning, I would look at the Disney map and plot out the day's events. Of course, I would take Steve and Lisa's requests and then plan our strategy to fit in as many sites as possible. Being in a wheelchair was a definite bonus. There were separate entrances for wheelers at each venue, and there was hardly ever a line! It was so much fun!

The second trip was also to Florida, but in December with my aide Floe. St. Louis had a ton of snow on the ground. Our 5:30 p.m. plane was delayed.

Steve, Floe, and I used the airport's family bathroom with a lockable door to do my cath. This is a private bathroom used mostly by parents of small children with a plastic changing table in it. Well, I couldn't fit on that small table, so Steve and Floe transferred me to the floor, Floe cathed me, and they both put me back into my chair. Let me say, the floor of an airport bathroom is disgusting! (Thank God for the paper chucks pads that come in my cath kits.) After the cath, Floe said "It looks like we might be here for a while; I'm heading for the bar." I was a little put off by her announcing and doing this, but there wasn't too much to do while we waited for the weather to clear and our flight to depart. We waited and cathed every hour before our flight finally took off at 10:30 p.m. We landed in Orlando and picked up our rental van. We drove to Daytona Beach with Floe passed out in back, and we arrived at Steve's sister's house at 2:30 in the morning. Floe popped up with her hand on her forehead and said, "Are we there yet?" She was totally out of it. I soon learned that attendants, margaritas, and traveling don't mix well. I don't allow attendants to drink on the job now.

My third experience was flying down to Florida to catch a 7-day Caribbean cruise for a belated honeymoon. I brought an attendant with us, although she turned it into somewhat of a vacation for herself. I paid her, yet she would tell me what she would and would not do without consulting with Steve and me. The reservations got all mixed up, so the three of us had to share one room with a large closet area. So Steve, for the sake of privacy, slept in the closet. (God, I love him!) The cabin attendant thought we were strange when we asked for an extra mattress. But we made it work.

After 4 days, Steve and I asked my aide if we could have the room privately for a few hours. (She stayed in the cabin almost the whole trip.) But Steve and I needed some "alone time." We agreed upon a time for my aide to come back, but she came back early, ruining what little privacy Steve and I had. The last 2 days of our journey, my attendant was exhausted and slept for almost the rest of the trip. I think a full week of work was too much for her. Prior to this, she had only worked 6 hours a day, 5 days a week. Her job was to get me up in the morning (with a shower every other day) and do my cath at night. Other than that, she really just ate and slept.

Our plane landed in St. Louis and, as we waited outside the cockpit, I saw my electric wheelchair headed down the ramp toward me in a couple of pieces. I asked the staff why they took my chair apart. They said they thought I had acid batteries (most of the earlier electric chairs did, and the batteries had to be removed during travel because of possible spillage). But I had communicated to the airport staff in Florida that the chair had gel batteries so the batteries did not have to be removed. The airport staff had no answer. I then asked, "Who is going to put my chair together?" That's when my aide said, "Now calm down Katie. You know how testy you get." I was ready to fire her then and there, but I looked at Steve and we both knew we needed her to make it home, because her boyfriend was the one picking us up in my van. Well, the airport staff got my chair put back together and we were on our way. The whole ride home was silent. I'm sure my attendant's boyfriend was wondering what was up.

We got home and, later that day, I called and fired the very less-than-supportive attendant. I have also learned that when I fly, I put notices all over my wheelchair saying "This chair has gel batteries. Do not remove them."

One day, a different afternoon aide came into work and told me that her husband had to have her at home and she had to quit working for me. Man, I was so disappointed!

We worked great together. She had never worked with a person with a disability before but was really getting into it. Sometimes it seems like the really good attendants come and go so quickly.

I had one attendant who was very religious. When I asked her a question about her beliefs, she slapped me across the face. I sat there in disbelief. Aren't we all supposed to love everyone? For me, violence is not a way to bring me to your side.

Other attendant catastrophes include my van being backed into my house and breaking the rear window; a female attendant who was sexually attracted to me; attendants who read my personal mail and listened to my phone calls; and attendants who "borrowed" things without asking.

I had another attendant who was always sick and would not seek medical attention because she did not like taking medicine, which put my health in jeopardy. I had to let her go because of this, and she could not understand why.

I have noticed that some of my attendants have had issues with alcohol. My friends who use aides have experienced this issue as well. In the mid 1990s, my night aide reported for duty at 10 p.m. When she walked through the door, I could smell the liquor on her. I wanted to tell her to leave, but this was when I didn't have any back-up attendants available yet, and I really needed to empty my bladder then and there. I had nowhere to turn. My attendant did my transfer lift, and I barely landed in bed. Then she went into the kitchen to get a glass of water for my pills and *crash*, the glass broke. She came back to my room, and I asked her if she had been drinking. She fell to her knees and into my lap crying, saying how horrible her life was and that she didn't know what was wrong. I calmed her down, she dressed me for bed, and then she passed out in her bed. I don't think I slept at all that night. The next morning, I confronted her with what had happened the night before and she didn't remember any of it. As much as I really liked her, and still do today, I had to let her go.

I have had sheriffs and other police officials call me or stop by my home looking for former employees. Bail bondsmen, private detectives, and child-custody officials have called me as well. A former attendant was using my address for some of her bills. I quickly called the creditor and put a stop to that. Some still list me as their current employer years later! I can't believe the nerve of some people.

Finally, one of the things I can do for some of my attendants is to help them build their self-esteem. Many of the women I have met in this field have settled for less than they should have. The men and some of the children in their lives have taken advantage of them and/or verbally and physically abused them. Some of my attendants don't believe they have any worth. But because I am so motivated, it rubs off onto my attendants. The only problem with my empowering these women is that they improve themselves and move on to other jobs. Oh, well. I guess overall, it's a good thing.

So, to summarize, if you want to be a good attendant:

- Realize the importance of your job
- Keep your commitments
- Show up for your shift and be on time
- Respect your employer's body
- Respect your employer's home
- And ask yourself . . . "If I needed help, how would I like to be assisted?"

A PERSONAL CARE ATTENDANT'S PERSPECTIVES

I asked some of my current and former attendants to share their perspectives on attendant care and they responded to the following questions:

- How did you become interested in becoming a personal care attendant?
- What is your educational background and formal/informal training?
- What is your advice to others thinking about becoming a personal care attendant?
- What do you like about this type of occupation?
- What is the most important quality to carry into the job?
- Are there any humorous stories you can share?

Diane's Experiences

I have been an aide forever, but I'm not complaining because I love it. I cared for my grandmother with terminal cancer, my aunt with multiple sclerosis, my mother with Alzheimer's disease, and my father who had Parkinson's disease. I worked for a home health agency for 6 years and am currently doing private duty attendant care.

I am a high school graduate and have attended seminars, lectures, and workshops on CPR, Alzheimer's disease, dementia, stroke, and diabetes. I became an aide because I have a bubbly and humorous personality. My hope is that it will be contagious, and I can pass it on to those I'm helping. I'm at my fullest when I'm helping others.

My first caregiving experience was taking my grandmother to her radiation treatments. I listened to her and some of the other cancer patients. God blessed me with a personality to share with those in need. I feel other's emotional highs and lows. Their fear of death touched my heart. My guardian angels share in my efforts.

My care enables my clients to live as independently as possible. I feel as if I have contributed to their life in a small way. I can help give them a reason to smile. This work is often hard, and it won't make you rich, but it has other benefits and rewards. I can make a difference every day in the lives of those I assist.

The downside to assisting many elderly clients is their frailty, inactivity, and poor circulation. Often they "hibernate" from life and give up on physical activity. They become frustrated from lack of accomplishment. Therefore, I try to encourage my elderly clients by getting them washed and dressed and taking them out for a small errand or just for a drive. It's amazing to see them remembering what fun it is to get up and go somewhere! It just makes my day.

Other difficult issues include lack of family involvement. I'm amazed by the people who just "give up" and stop caring for the elder members of their family. I have also found that the elderly are often overmedicated and confused about their own medications.

The low pay for such a high-energy job can be a deterrent to becoming an aide. But I have learned how to juggle enough clients to keep my gas tank filled, keep food on the table, and live a very modest lifestyle.

Become an attendant if you have patience, patience, and more patience! You need to be a giver, not a taker. Sometimes you may have to work weekends and/or holidays as an aide. You need to be a reliable person, not only when you "want to," but each day you have committed to work. The elderly need consistent, dependable, and reliable attendant care.

Finally, respect the natural aging process. There are some things you can control in life and others you cannot. Aging is the latter. So care about the senior members in your life. After all, you may need help in your golden years!

Tracy's Experiences

In addition to working with Katie in the mornings, I have worked with elderly women who have a wide range of physical and cognitive limitations as a result of Alzheimer's disease or stroke-related dementia, assisting with all kinds of personal care and activities of daily living. I have never worked for an agency or skilled nursing facility because I prefer to work directly for individuals and their families, focusing entirely on in-home care and private duty in nursing facilities. This allows me the maximum freedom and opportunity to provide patients with the best and most personalized care possible.

I have been a personal care attendant for 8 years. I have no certifications or formal training in the health field whatsoever. Everything I know I have learned from patients, their families, other caregivers, personal research, and good old-fashioned trial-and-error. All it takes is patience and a willingness to learn, coupled with empathy and compassion.

I became a personal care attendant because of my great-grandmother. I was lucky enough to have Gram in my life until I was 19, when I watched her die a slow and painful death from cancer that spread to nearly all of her vital organs. I wanted desperately to care for her myself, but I had neither the knowledge nor the experience to do so. I was totally helpless as I watched her suffer a horrible death that could have been more peaceful if she had been properly medicated and cared for.

Knowing what I do now, I realize that it happened that way because my family lacked knowledge, resources, and experience in dealing with her illness. At the time, I just wanted to make sure that the same thing didn't happen to other people's parents and grandparents.

Right after Gram died, an LPN friend of mine who worked for an Adult Day Care program was overwhelmed with requests for evening and weekend help, so she asked me to help out with some of the lighter cases. She gave me some very basic training, and I started out on an as-needed basis with women who had early-onset Alzheimer's disease but were still physically strong. Six months later, I accepted a regular job with Rose, a sweet and spunky 81-year-old woman who had mobility limitations and mild dementia due to multiple "mini-strokes." I ended up caring for Rose until her death 6 years later, learning the things I needed to know about caregiving along the way as her needs increased. I felt that I was caring for my great-grandmother vicariously through caring for Rose and all my other "ladies." I was able to provide them and their families with the kind of care and advocacy that my Gram should have had.

When assisting a person with a disability, the most important things are communication, communication, and communication. Did I mention communication? It is vital for the individual to clearly and specifically ask for what they want and need. Even if the individual has lost the ability to communicate, communication is still possible with those family members who know them best.

My philosophy as a caregiver is simply this— "Anything you want, you got it." I believe that people should basically have things done the way they want. If it is safe, legal, and within my physical capability, I'll do it. I do not believe in imposing my will, opinions, or attitudes upon an individual who has already lost enough of her independence.

In order for this to happen, however, the individual (or family members) must state their needs explicitly, which also includes constructive criticism. If something isn't done the way you want it done, don't be afraid to speak up. I have to know your wishes in order to fulfill them. By the same token, it is always helpful to hear about the things you are doing right. Everyone deserves praise and appreciation for what they do well. This tends to increase confidence, responsibility, and loyalty—qualities you want to encourage in your personal care attendant.

In addition, communication is a two-way street. The caregiver must also be open and unafraid to articulate her questions, concerns, and suggestions in order to provide the best care possible. I treat my patients with respect, consideration, and the utmost concern for their welfare, and I like to be treated the same way. The bottom line is: When these things run both ways, everybody receives the maximum benefit.

The best thing about doing this type of work is the people. I have been blessed to work with the most amazing and extraordinary individuals and their families. One of the questions I am asked most often is, "Isn't it hard because you get close to people and then they die?" My answer is always the same: Of course it's hard to lose people, but the best part is being close to them and their families. You cannot be someone's personal care attendant for any length of time and not develop some kind of personal relationship with them. If you can, then this business is not for you. A certain amount of emotional compartmentalization is necessary to get the job done, but the best part is sharing laughs, triumphs, tears, and losses. This is what compassion is about—sharing our humanity with each other.

Second only to the wonderful people I am privileged to work with is the knowledge that I am making a difference in someone's life and the lives of their families. Everyone has heard terrible stories of abuse, neglect, and substandard care. It is immensely rewarding to know that I am providing the absolute best care possible and that patients and their families can breathe easier knowing they have someone dependable and trustworthy to rely on, who has their best interest at heart. When one has all the worries and hassles that come with disability and illness, a little peace of mind is priceless.

There can be many frustrating aspects to being an aide. The absolute worst is dealing with families who are only interested in providing minimal care for patients, and family members who are not diligent in providing basic care necessities. As an aide, you have to contend with the fact that you are not ultimately responsible for the patient—the patient or their family members are. You cannot make medical care decisions for them. Instead, you have to respect their wishes and decisions, even if you do not agree or approve, and do the best for them you can.

The key to becoming a first-rate personal care attendant is to put yourself in the other person's position. Ask yourself, "If this were me, how would I want to be treated? What would be my biggest concerns? What would I want and need?" When you constantly ask such questions, you increase your awareness and perspective and, as you gain experience, this makes you better at your job. It is also invaluable in combating frustration and burnout.

One of the most frequent comments I hear when I tell people what I do is, "I could never do that." While there are certainly people who can't and shouldn't do this type of work, my guess is that most people can. It just takes a positive attitude and genuine concern for another person's well-being. Anyone who is considering this kind of work should know that it requires patience and compassion. If you think being a personal care attendant is like working in retail or at fast food restaurants, look elsewhere. If you are honest, dependable, willing to learn, and want to make a difference in the world through helping people, we need *you* in this line of work.

Lisa's Experiences

I had never been a personal care attendant before I started assisting Katie at night, off and on for almost 10 years. I obtained my degree in psychology, took some continuing education classes in the arts, and put in

3 years as a social worker. Then I got a Missouri Aesthetician License. I consider this to be in the health field because teaching people how to care for their skin is good for the body, mind, and spirit.

I considered becoming an attendant to see how I would deal with someone who is paralyzed. When I responded to Katie's classified ad and heard her voice over the phone, full of determination, with an amazing attitude, I thought to myself, "This could be someone I could learn something from."

When assisting a person with a disability, communication is number one. That is closely followed by respect and bonding. To me, it's a working respectable friendship with a strong bonding opportunity. This type of work is personal—undressing, dressing, cathing, changing tampons, and cleaning up the occasional bladder and bowel accidents. So both sides better know how to communicate with each other.

Speaking of communication, when I came into her room in the middle of the night to empty her bladder, it was always an adventure. Many times she was awake, but then there were nights she was half asleep and babbling on and on about something or barking orders that could not be deciphered! I called it my "cath time entertainment!"

What I liked most about the job was spending time talking, laughing, and crying about life. What I didn't like were the times Katie's "perfectionist" attitude frustrated me, although if I were in her shoes, I would like things done a certain way, too.

To do this type of work, you have to have a genuinely kind and caring heart. There also has to be a "click" between both individuals. If you are unhappy or depressed, I don't think this is a job for you. If you want to do this work badly enough, and it is meant for you at the time, a special person will come into your life. Also, don't be embarrassed or upset when the person you are assisting throws up, poops, or pees on herself.

Just do the job of cleaning them up and act like it's no big thing. Just try to put yourself in her place. Whenever these things happen, take a deep breath and say to yourself "I hope there is someone to take care of me when I get this way!"

Bethany's Experiences

I met Katie and her husband Steve when I became their massage therapist a few years ago. I have only worked one job as a personal care attendant, for a gentleman approximately 70 years old who was diagnosed with the beginning stages of Parkinson's disease. I have no formal training but I have personal life experiences that qualified me for this type of work.

I have had many different jobs in the past: restaurant work, a job in an office, and in real estate. I quickly learned that the office atmosphere was not where I wanted to be. I wanted to do something more humanitarian. I looked into the Peace Corps, but that didn't work out as I had hoped. That's when I began researching naturopathic medicine, which led me to massage therapy.

I'd been practicing massage for almost 3 years and was beginning to feel the wear and tear on my hands when I was approached with an opportunity to supplement my income as an aide. The job was described as "helping out an elderly fellow who was a professor and a photographer during his working years." I found him to be incredibly interesting and wise as a person. He had full function of his body, but every once in a while he would lose his balance and fall due to his Parkinson's disease.

His family felt more comfortable having an assistant around the house to see after him, as opposed to having a hired nurse. They felt that a nurse would give the impression that he was sick, and they wanted more of a companion for him. It seemed to be the perfect combination, and it was an opportunity for me to learn something new from an amazing person. Hopefully, I was interesting and caring enough to keep him occupied mentally as well as spiritually. Our working relationship lasted 8 months.

When working with anyone, regardless of a "labeled disability," it's important to have respect and trust for the person you're assisting. The relationship between a person with a disability and the assistant is incredibly important because of the "vulnerability factor." A wide range of emotions is shared between the two that are not usually displayed in any other work environment.

The person with the disability is dealing with emotions on a different level from what is going on in the rest of so-called normal society. Their daily existence presents different challenges. The best-case scenario for everyone is to check egos at the door. Many times, that doesn't happen. There also needs to be an understanding of boundaries—exactly what is expected from the personal care attendant and what is not acceptable. Nothing, if at all possible, should be assumed.

I love the freedom of this type of work. To some, it may not seem like freedom. To me, it frees me from an office and punching in and out on a time clock. I am able to be out in the world interacting with people, experiencing real emotions, and not hiding behind office politics. That doesn't mean I don't have to meet expectations of professionalism. If the right attendant partnership is formed, and I am allowed to be myself, it's wonderful work. I also think it is a gift to learn from the wisdom of another person's life experiences different from my own.

Honestly, what frustrates me most is when I realize I am spending too much time taking care of another person's needs and slacking on my own. I begin to feel resentful over the slightest of duties. Balance is a challenge.

The standards of hiring in this type of job are different from any other. This is a time to use intuition. Know your commitments—children, second or third jobs, and schooling. Also remember, in most cases, that you are not working just with a person you are assisting, but with their entire family. Know your boundaries with each family member. Be sure you have enough time in your schedule to take care of your client's needs as well as your own. Finally, drop all expectations of what you think a person with a disability is like.

Rhonda's Experiences

I have been an overnight attendant for Katie on and off for over 4 years. My prior work experience included 12 years as a veterinary technician. While I had no experience in the field as an aide, after answering Katie's ad and meeting her, I thought "Why not?" I soon learned that being helpful and making Katie's life a little easier made the work worth the effort. And getting paid for it was cool, too.

I did have two areas of concern. The first was that I needed patience from Katie because I can sometimes be forgetful, especially in learning new things. But I quickly learned how to transfer her with ease and then mastered the ability to cath her after her other attendants and her husband trained me.

My only other concern is an ongoing fear that I might not wake up in the middle of the night to cath Katie. Lucky for me, Katie's voice is far from paralyzed! Also, we always set an alarm in Katie's room to wake us both. Many times I have heard the alarm go off and have come in to cath Katie and she's still sound asleep! Then I just go about my duties and back to bed until we have to get up in the morning.

The best piece of advice I can offer those wanting to be an aide is to treat the people you are assisting the way you like to be treated. Also, if you don't have any experience, don't worry. Work with your employer and figure it out. Just go for it!

Mike's Experiences

I'm 39 years old, and I became an attendant when a neighbor asked me to help him with some of the things he wanted to do. I also entered the field to make some extra money and hopefully learn something new. Becoming a personal care attendant has given me great satisfaction.

I am a person with a disability, but my disability hasn't hindered my physical abilities. My disability is more of a learning disability. Reading, writing, and spelling challenge me on a regular basis. I'm not stupid. But processing and understanding numbers and letters may take me longer than it does the average person.

I have a bachelor's degree in health, an associate's degree as a physical therapist assistant, and an associate's degree in speech communication. I also participated in the sport of wrestling. Who knew that would serve me and the people I now lift so well!

My dad was a physical education teacher for 38 years. My first experience in meeting people who were labeled "handicapped" happened when my father developed an adaptive recreation room at local junior high school. I helped him set up activities so that students of any ability could experience some form of physical fitness.

Later in life, some friends of mine started a travel group called Adventures for All. With the help of this group, I developed a program called "Fishing with Mike," which consisted of a 3-day camping and fishing experience.

A person in need is my ideal client. We all need help in some way. And if you are considering the attendant care field as an occupation, I say Fantastic! Terrific! Great! We need more people like you. Especially you guys out there. We need more men in this field.

My advice on how to conduct oneself as a professional in the work place has four basic components: 1) Know your role; 2) know yourself; 3) be yourself; and 4) have fun.

One of the scariest attendant care experiences I've ever had happened on New Years Eve 1999. I was with my friends at an Adventures for All outing. We started the night at a movie theater. When the movie was over, we came out of the theater and there was snow everywhere, and lots of it. Several people in our group used wheelchairs, but the walks and curb cuts were very slippery. So the plan was to assist the people in chairs, one at a time, and load them into our van. One of our friends riding in a power chair didn't see the edge of the curb and, while turning around, one of his wheels fell off the curb and he and his chair flipped over. He hit his head on the parking lot, and I went after him. I got his wheelchair upright and lifted him back into his chair. Then we all noticed a large golf ball-size lump on his head. We gathered up a bunch of snow, put it in a plastic bag, and put it on the lump on his forehead as we headed for the hospital. As it turned out, there was no permanent damage. But it was stressful way to start the New Year!

The word *interdependence* is a word I learned from a friend that describes a community in which people share their particular strengths with one another in order to make up for and eliminate the weakness we all possess.

The people who want to make a difference in this world by strengthening themselves and those around them are those who are willing to share what they have. They are the purveyors of the interdependence movement. People are willing to give and take, until our needs do not exist. A personal care attendant can do that every day!

IN CONCLUSION

The following chapters give caregiving tips from a spouse, a child, and an aide of an elderly person. So many common denominators exist in caring for anyone, but I think you'll enjoy these enlightening perspectives.

CHAPTER 5

WHEN THE CAREGIVER IS A SPOUSE OR SIGNIFICANT OTHER

There is a federal law that offers some support for working caregivers through the Family and Medical Leave Act (FMLA). This allows eligible workers up to 12 weeks a year of unpaid leave for family caregiving without loss of job security or health benefits. Although valuable, FMLA does not help those who cannot afford to take unpaid leave. Also, restrictions such as company size and the amount of time a worker has been employed keep many people from being covered.

This chapter discusses the issues of spouses or partners caring for a significant other who has a disability. It will also touch on when additional attendant care in your own home may be necessary. My husband Steve wrote the following on being a caregiver.

I met Katie almost 3 years after her injury. I was a program manager and supervisor of independent living specialists at Services for Independent Living in Columbia, Missouri. The day was February 1, 1993, and our staff escorted several of our consumers with various disabilities to our state capitol in Jefferson City to educate state representatives and senators about the needs of people with disabilities (PWD). Our consumers were there to testify before the House Appropriations Committee to request funding increases for the state PCA (personal care attendant) program. This general revenue–funded program allowed PWDs to hire their own personal care attendants and live in their own homes, instead of a nursing home or other institutionalized setting. You can read more about our courtship and life together in Chapter 9, About the Author.

After that first meeting, Katie and I spent the next 6 years getting to know each other. I made the 2-hour trip to St. Louis on a regular basis. I wanted an intimate relationship soon after we started seeing each other every weekend, but she wasn't ready. So I gave up hoping to have Katie as a girlfriend and just enjoyed a friendship. It was tough, but a year and a half later, I got a kiss! It was so worth the wait. Being best friends first created the best relationship I've ever been in.

Soon after we were dating exclusively, Katie asked her overnight attendant, Lisa, to show me her catheterization (cath) procedure, which made sense to me. I was now able to cath her and provide whatever care she needed, which allowed the two of us to travel together and/or just spend more time together uninterrupted.

On May 27, 2000, we were able to marry without fear of my income kicking Katie off her Social Security and Medicaid. Katie received a modest settlement from an auto manufacturer in 1999. We could officially continue our fun and fantastic life together.

I knew what I was getting into when we married. I was prepared to love, honor, cherish, cath every 5 hours, and perform additional duties as needed. I had no doubts about my desire to become Katie's husband and care-partner, and I have no regrets now. I enjoy assisting my wife with her personal care as well as helping her run our business, Access-4-All, Inc.

I am also aware of issues facing care-partners, whose spouse or significant other may incur a disabling condition after they had been in relationships for many years. Through my 13-year experience at Services for Independent Living in Columbia, Missouri, as well as my 18-month stint at the National Multiple Sclerosis (MS) Society Gateway Area Chapter in St. Louis, I have worked with dozens of families who had to deal with the issue of a spouse becoming a caregiver.

I also worked with individuals who were newly injured and their families, helping them decide what would be the best attendant care route to take for their situation. I helped develop a personal care attendant training program in Columbia, in addition to assisting in the development of a multiagency assisted living home in Hermann, Missouri. This home helped several men with cerebral palsy to live independently with managed attendant care. At the MS Society, I supported self-help groups and I facilitated the Care-partner Reprieve group for the care-partners of people with MS.

What works for Katie and me is mainly that we love each other. Yes, we argue on occasion, but we have a deep love base that keeps us happy. We have a mix of me aiding Katie every afternoon and providing her overnight care Friday and Saturday each week. We hire personal care attendants to help her in the mornings, and an overnight attendant comes to our aid Sunday through Thursdays. I'm a night owl, so I can run my errands after our night attendant arrives. This mix has worked well for us.

When the spouse is the sole care provider, a loving relationship is essential. I have met several families where the spouse provided one-hundred percent of care. I have seen this in a positive light more than in a negative light. Many people don't want to invite strangers into their homes, or can't afford to pay for outside assistance. However, it is important for the caregiver to try to find others to assist from time to time, such as when the care-partner has a doctor's appointment or needs a break. No one can do everything. Learn to ask for help when you need it.

Often, respite can be provided by other family members, neighbors with nursing/LPN backgrounds, or home health agencies. *Respite* is basically the ability for a care-partner to get some time off from being the sole care provider. As long as a loving relationship exists and the care-partner can get occasional respite, this caregiving spouse situation can work quite well.

There are ways to make the attendant care provision fun with your spouse. For example, if your spouse needs assistance with a shower, by all means get naked with her or him! It's fun to be intimate, plus it's a good way to keep from getting too hot or getting your clothes soaked. Live it up! This is your beloved, remember? People with disabilities are still sexual beings with all the "normal" earthly desires.

Have fun! Make bathing, dressing, feeding, driving, and caring for another a labor of love. Its cold comfort but, what if the roles were reversed? Think about the care you would want, and then give it to one needing it.

Enjoy your caregiving as the special event it happily is. You are helping your loved one live as independently and as happily as possible. Pat yourself on the back for being a great person!!!

Show compassion and kindness to your loved one, and you will receive appreciation in return. (Unless he or she is perpetually grumpy—that is a whole challenge in itself.)

DEALING WITH FRUSTRATION

To be honest, there will be times when providing care to your spouse isn't easy. As a human being, you will get frustrated from time to time. If either of you are in a bad mood, if one of you is ill, if you had plans but your respite backs out or your regular personal care attendant cancels on you, frustration will rear its head. Regardless of the situation, you must do your best to remember that you love this person. Work from your heart, your love, and your light. Focus and breathe in from your nose and out through your mouth—this is the breathing technique humans are supposed to use anyway to achieve maximum energy. Repeatedly take long, slow inhales through your nose and exhale via your mouth—this will calm down angry feelings and positively energize you at the same time. Vocal toning can be helpful as well, to release feelings of frustration. A good shout can do wonders. But be careful where you do this. You don't want to scare the neighbors!

Discuss any concerns you have regarding attendant care openly with your spouse, such as scheduling, duties, or time off. If you have been assisting your spouse with cooking, cleaning, and other household chores, and you need to rest, be sure to ask your loved one if he needs anything before you sit down. Learn how to find your own space in your home, one that is just yours for relaxing, watching TV/listening to music, meditating, reading, working on the computer, playing games, or other leisure activities. Be sure to discuss boundaries with your spouse regarding your need for time and space for you. It's about compromise. Make time for yourself while remembering the commitments you made to be a spouse, for better or worse. Choose to make it better yourself.

Ultimately, work from the realization that as humans, our souls are all one, playing God's game of life on this planet. As we open our hearts to others and share our love and light freely, we help all of humanity as well as the Earth evolve and grow. The acquisition of disabling conditions does not mean life is over—far from it! With love and support from family and friends, PWDs can and do live exciting and happy lives.

Your path is to assist your loved one. But again, if you need help, ask for it! Don't be shy. Ask other family members, friends, church members, coworkers (as appropriate), or others who might want to volunteer. If you hire personal care attendants and are concerned about your spouse's safety as well as your belongings, you don't have to leave the house. Instead, go to "your space" while others are providing care for your spouse. Relax, read, recreate indoors, and enjoy your time off in your own way.

You will need to find a way to be a successful care-partner; one who can enjoy helping your spouse, and one with the ability to request outside assistance as needed. Keep yourself happy, healthy, and physically able. Keep yourself in shape by exercising a few times a week. Walk, lift weights, put on an exercise video, or take a fitness class. The better shape you're in, the more strength and stamina you have to care for someone else.

Helping others can be extremely rewarding. Find the beauty of providing assistance to others.

Recognize yourself to be the true "Angel on Earth" that you become when you agree to provide loving assistance to one another. Be the best person you can be. Love yourself, love your spouse, and live your lives together happily ever after.

-Steve Banister

In the next chapter, we'll look at caring for children with disabilities.

CHAPTER 6

CARING FOR CHILDREN WITH DISABILITIES

Although there are many similarities between caring for a child and helping an adult or elderly person with a disability, I met a young person who wanted to share his perspective. He has some great advice on assisting kids with disabilities. (Some information has been changed to protect this person's privacy.)

A friend introduced me to an administrative staff member of a pediatric facility in a rural Illinois town. She introduced me to a feisty, fun, and intelligent 13-year-old boy who lived at this pediatric facility. I will call him Joe. I met with Joe after his school day, and was accompanied by a very cool therapist named Sam. Sam is a paraplegic and uses a manual wheelchair. I really liked Sam's can-do attitude, and he had definitely earned Joe's respect. Sam and my husband Steve also joined in on the conversation. I really thought I was going to need a lot of Sam's help to communicate with Joe, because Joe has cerebral palsy and is unable to speak, other than making a general sound of agreement or disagreement. He communicates using a sheet of paper with the letters of the alphabet on it. He bends forward using his nose to spell out each word he wants to share. It's a slow and steady way for him to communicate, but after watching Sam talk to Joe, I was soon able to follow along too. This middle school student is reading on a high school level, so expressing his thoughts was a piece of cake. Joe told me that someday I'll be reading *his* book. I can't wait!

Joe is wise beyond his years on our planet. Early on, his home life wasn't ideal. His natural family couldn't meet all of his needs and, about a year ago, he came to reside at the pediatric facility. It's not the living situation Joe really wants, but it is going to have to do for now. I'm sure every one of the children living in that facility wishes to be with their natural parents instead. But, in many cases, they have physical, emotional, and psychological needs that their natural parents can't take care of. In some cases, parents have neglected their child's needs or have physically or emotionally abused them. Finally, some of these kids have aging parents who are physically unable to care for their children. Many of these parents give up their parental rights, some willingly and some who are legally made to do so. All of this is to ensure that kids with disabilities get the care they need.

A variety of "home-away-from-home" settings are available today. You can find them through your state Department of Mental Health and/or Department of Child Services. I did a "Google" search on the Internet and typed in "Children's Homes" and my state and got info on all kinds of places. In Missouri, our Regional Centers have this information.

Here are some things Joe wants people to remember:

- Children need to be loved.
- Children have feelings too.

- When new aides come to help, they really
  need to know and understand what a
  child is capable of doing. Talk to the child
  first. Get to know him.
- It is important to be sensitive and gentle
  when working with children.
- Fun is a must for any kid! Make time to
  play on a regular basis.
- Don't fuss over children all the time. Let
  kids be kids. Love them but give them
  some space too!
- Let a child make a mistake, and don't yell
  at her.
- Most importantly, children, regardless of
  their ability level, deserve respect. You
  can't expect to get it if you don't give it.

Joe is one cool kid and is a shining example of the
motto "Life Goes On!"

Sam gave me his list of suggestions too! Here is what
he wants you to know:

- Keep in mind that the cognitive ability
  does not always match up with physical
  ability. You cannot be one-hundred percent
  sure of what a child does or does not understand. It is very degrading when you
  talk down to a child who knows what's
  going on. So, communicate. Talk *and* listen.
- Remember that you are working with a
  child. All children have special concerns,
  problems, and issues that go hand in hand
  with being a kid. Having a disability
  doesn't make a child exempt from the situations that take place as a person grows up.
- Play with your child. Two hopeful goals
  in childhood are to play and learn about
  the world. Help your children experience

and accomplish these goals. Possess the ability to have fun and actively assist your child in doing so. There is more to life than popping in a video. Get out and do something!

- Assist children in being as successful as they can be. Help them create personal, academic, and other goals for themselves, and encourage them to complete them and do more. See a future for every child. Goals can include being able to communicate independently, dressing themselves, being able to instruct others on how to care for them, or learning positive ways to deal with negative feelings. All this will foster self-esteem in a child with a disability—or any child for that matter.

- Encourage independence. Adults often do too much for their children. This is even more prevalent when it comes to kids with disabilities. It's important to let children do anything they can on their own, starting early in life. Adults need to avoid encouraging "learned helplessness" in any child. Help your child empower herself. Sure, it may take more time at first, but practicing independence can become easier with time.

- Regarding a child's privacy, sometimes your best tool is common sense. Do you want the whole world knowing your private issues? Do you want others watching you empty your bladder, complete your bowel routine, or take a bath? I don't think so. So, respect a child's privacy. Don't discuss a child's diagnosis or special needs with just anyone. Keep client information confidential. It's their business and their decision to share. And, please, respect a child's body by covering up personal body parts. Also, don't forget to shut the bathroom or bedroom door during bathing and dressing times.

- When it comes to working with adolescents, teens with disabilities experience the same issues as their peers without disabilities do. All teenagers struggle with hormones and identity issues. They are trying to establish "Who am I?" Be patient with them. Help them find appropriate ways to deal with identity struggles. Try talking to them about these feelings and about the changes their bodies are undergoing. If you can't, find a counselor, family member, or friend who can.

- It's all about balance. When it comes to working with children with disabilities, demanding expectations don't really work. On the other hand, letting your child have a pity party every day is just as unproductive. Establish goals, expect success, and be patient if it takes a while to accomplish these goals. You can be firm and loving at the same time.

As I ended my visit with Joe and Sam, we had a few final thoughts:

- Remember that life should be fun. Yes, living with a disability is hard work, but try and find joy in each and every day. Go fishing, take a walk or roll around the neighborhood, or go to the park. Kids are kids no matter their ability, and fun should be a part of their daily lives.
- Let children be their own person.

- Create a helpful child and avoid the path of helplessness.
- Instill respect and it will come back to you.
- Expect a child with a disability to act as appropriately as their peers without disabilities do. Remind them of their age and their expected behavior.

I leave you with Joe's final thought . . .

Remember
that no matter
how disabled
someone is
there is
a whole person
inside of him.

The next chapter explores the specials needs of the elderly disabled.

CHAPTER 7

THE AGING PROCESS AND CARING FOR THE ELDERLY

Aging isn't easy for anyone. It was difficult to see my father pass away in 1998, but he put up one hell of a fight. His asthma slowed him down, and his heart finally gave out. But he kept going and doing, right up to the end. A few years later, my mother had knee surgery that developed complications. We also think she had a small stroke while in the hospital undergoing treatment for myasthenia gravis, but that wasn't medically proven. She recognizes the fact that her short-term memory is going.

It's been difficult for her, but she's still living in her own home with the help of one of my older brothers. Currently, she has an aide come in to help with personal care, but her losses are great, and her limitations keep her inside most of the time. Some of my family members commit to having dinner with her once a week, and we take her out to hear music and visit the bookstore and department stores. She loves reading and short trips to get out and about.

Assisting the elderly is different from helping a young person with a spinal cord injury. The elderly often need assistance due to physical loss, limited mobility, incontinence, short-term memory loss, dementia, Alzheimer's disease, and other illnesses that affect one's mind and the ability to care for oneself. But also keep in mind that, as people age, their bodies may become frail but their minds may still be functioning normally.

People who are elderly need a caring person to help them at this stage in their life. It's often the daughters in the family who assume this role. This fact disappoints me, but it's true.

One of my mother's favorite attendants, Diane, gave me a wonderful list of tips on how to care for the elderly.

- You must understand that there are some things you can't control in life, and the aging process is one of them. If we are fortunate, we all grow old. Although there are steps you can take to make the process healthier, such as eating right, exercising, and not smoking, sooner or later, we all leave our current physical existence.
- Treat the elderly as you want to be treated, at any age. Avoid the tendency to treat older people as if they were infants! Instead, help them keep their dignity by treating them with respect.
- Be creative. Find new things to do. Break out of old habits.
- Be positive. No one wants to hang out with someone who always sees the glass as half empty. Yes, bad things happen every day. But remember, what you think creates your reality. Be careful with your thoughts, because they just might come true!
- Leave your personal problems elsewhere. Attend to your client. Chances are that your aging parent or client won't be able to solve your problems. They're dealing with enough already.

- If it is at all possible, take your aging family members out on a regular basis. Going to a park or out to lunch can make a world of difference in attitude for a person who may spend a lot of time indoors.
- As we age, it doesn't mean that a person has stopped liking everything. Find something that brings a smile to another's face. Maybe it's a favorite movie, book, or food. Maybe it's taking a drive to a favorite spot or place from the past.
- Dress your aging clients in bright and attractive clothes, do their hair, put on some lipstick, put on a hat and a necktie. We all want to look good. When you look good, you feel good.
- Help them remember their favorite things, childhood memories, their former occupations. Ask them about the past. Pull out the pictures and albums. If they don't have a book of memories, help them make one!
- Actions often speak louder than words. If you have children of your own, it's important that they see that you respect your own parents. Live as an example. With time, you're going to grow old too, and you may be in need of assistance. To paraphrase an old song, "Teach your children well!"
- Accept the fact that a role reversal often happens as your parents begin to age. You, the child, become the parent when it comes to making life decisions for those who can no longer make such decisions for themselves. These issues include driving a vehicle, home maintenance, health care, medications, and managing finances.
- Use your resources. There are all kinds of places to find information, such as the Alzheimer's Association, the Department

of Health and Human Services, and the Department of Aging. Use a computer's search engine like Google and type in "elderly care" or "elder care" to find all kinds of websites and articles.

- Make time to spend with your elders: Don't just "stick them" someplace and forget about them. On the other hand, don't become a slave to your aging parents, and remember to encourage them to do as much for themselves as possible. Again, the importance of finding balance pops up.
- Remember—life doesn't stop until you take your last breath. So why not enjoy life as much as possible? Take time to smell the flowers and—while you're at it—bring your aging friends along for the ride, too!

A last note . . .

Before I decided to write this guide, I had to research what was already published. Currently, the majority of caregiving books focus on caring for the elderly population. If you provide or supervise the care for an older adult and you want more specific information, go to a book-selling website or your local bookstore, and search "caregiving" books. I found helpful guides that have been published in the last 4 or 5 years.

Some of these books address financial management, living wills, power of attorney authorizations, emergency alert systems, diet, health maintenance, insurance, driving skills, exercise, medications, and other areas of concern regarding our aging citizens.

CHAPTER 8

ATTENDANT CARE—
WHAT A SCARE

The following was written as a result of my search for attendants after placing an ad in the help wanted section of my local newspaper. A friend of mine came over for lunch one day and listened in on the phone calls I received in response to the ad (I use a speaker phone for ease). I promise you, these are honest-to-goodness conversations I've had with the people who called. I may have changed a few things to protect the innocent, but you'll get the idea.

It's OK to laugh and enjoy this section. After 16 years of living a life as a woman on wheels, I've learned that laughing is essential, and you can't take the process personally. And that goes double for when it comes to managing your own personal care. You need to face the fact that people are the way they are, laugh about it, and go on.

I turned this story into a performance piece while I was a founding performance member of the disAbility Project (the A is capitalized because the project focuses on abilities) in St. Louis, Missouri. To find out more about this theater troupe, go to their website at www.DisabilityProject.com.

So please, enjoy . . .

Over the years I have been fortunate enough to find friends who share the same type of dependency on others as I do. We all have our own personal care attendant "horror" stories.

Molly is a friend and paraplegic, paralyzed from the waist down, who likes hanging out. We both like pizza, movies, and having fun. We both see our disabilities as difficult circumstances, but we use a lot of humor to overcome them.

One afternoon during the early days of living independently, Molly came over for lunch. Molly drives a beautiful two-door red sports car with a car topper on it. A car topper is a storage space on the roof of a car, with a mechanism that lowers, raises, and stores her folded manual wheelchair while she drives. She rolled through my door saying, "Hey! What's up?"

"Not me!" I answered as I rolled over to greet her.

She continued with an attempt to make me laugh, "Why, you look lower than a snake's front belt buckle!" It did make me smile. I told Molly that my morning attendant had quit last Friday without any notice and that I was stuck in bed for the whole day until my afternoon aide came in at 3 p.m. Molly rolled into the kitchen to help herself to a glass of water saying, "Well that sucks!"

I agreed with her, and told her I had already put an ad in the paper. I felt that someone was bound to call. The economy was a little sluggish, and a lot of people were looking for a job. I just needed to find someone and find that person soon!

Molly sympathized and asked if she could do anything. Then the phone rang. I invited Molly to listen in, and I hit the speaker phone button.

I said, "Hello?" There was no response. I said again, "Hello?"

Finally, after what seemed an hour, a soft voice answered, "Hello, can you hear me? Hello? Hold on. Wait a minute. Wait a minute. Now let me turn down my TV. There, now."

Through all the rambling, I said with a loud voice, "HELLO!"

The caller snapped back with, "Look honey. You don't have to shout. I'm not deaf."

I couldn't help but be polite saying, "Oh, I'm sorry." Then the voice said, "I'm calling about the ad in the paper."

"Fantastic. I have a few questions for you." I looked at Molly who was listening in with me.

"Yes, yes, go on," the caller replied.

"I was wondering, can you transfer and lift 129 pounds?" I asked.

"Oh my, heavens, no! I'm 97 years old! I can't do that. But good luck to you sweetie!" I hit my speaker button off and Molly laughed.

She asked, "Are all your calls like that?"

"Just about!" I responded. Then the phone rang again. "Cool. Another call."

"Go for it!" encouraged Molly.

"Hello?" I said.

"I am calling about the ad, and I am what you're looking for!" said the loud booming voice on the other end.

"Well," I said, "let me . . . ," and I was quickly cut off by the caller.

"I have great references. You could talk to Miss Jones. I took care of her poor sickly little girl. Lord, it was a blessing when that little girl died." Molly and I looked at each other in disbelief over what this woman was saying. The caller continued, "So I'm available now!"

"Well," I said, "I'm looking for someone who will. . . ."

"Be on time," she answered and continued with, "Oh, that's me! Except for Thursdays, no wait, Fridays. No. No. It is Thursdays. Yes. Yes. That's it. It is Thursdays. No, no . . . Well, never mind. I have paper and pen in hand as we speak. Where do you live? I could come over right . . . now!"

"Well, I hear someone at my door. I need to get going, but thanks for calling!" I said and ended the call.

"Man, she wore me out!" said Molly.

I answered, "While it's another example of independent living being a challenge, it sure beats a nursing home!"

Molly shared a somewhat similar story to me about her niece, Kelly. Kelly has multiple sclerosis and also lives with the help of attendants. One morning her attendant, Helga, got quite a surprise! Helga boomed through Kelly's front door with her "rise and shine" attitude. Kelly still had "sleep" in her eyes noting it was 6:30 in the morning, and Helga wasn't due to come in until 10:30. Helga said she had things to do but Kelly quickly reminded her that she was the one who paid her. Helga was oblivious.

Then Helga pulled back Kelly's sheets and out jumped David, Kelly's boyfriend! David leaped from the bed and ran out the door saying, "I'll call you later!"

Helga freaked and said, "Well . . . I never! I demand an explanation!"

"Well, David and I have been dating for 2 years and . . . ," Kelly tried to answer. but Helga cut her off, feeling repulsed by the whole situation. Kelly had had enough and told Helga to leave and never come back. Kelly can do most of her care on her own but needs an attendant for her showers and help around the house.

At the end of Molly's story I said, "Now *that's* an aide from *hell*!!!"

Then I shared my aide-from-hell story with Molly. I was waiting for one of my attendants to arrive for her shift one afternoon, thinking "Where is she? She's over an hour late. My bladder is going to explode!"

In rushed my attendant Mary, saying, "Oh, I'm so sorry I'm late. But you'll never *believe* what happened to me."

"Well, I can only imagine," I was thinking to myself.

Mary went on to say, "My car wouldn't start. so I called AAA. It took them an hour to get there. As the mechanic was working on my car, my husband, Rosco showed up, drunk as a skunk and started a fight with him. Well, the neighbors came out and everyone was screaming and cheering. Then, out of nowhere, a news van drove by, and a reporter jumped out and started filming. Naturally, I was so excited. I had never been on TV before! The next moment, the cops showed up and took Rosco away. My car was finally fixed and that was why I am late."

I screamed, "This is the third time you've been late this week, and it's only Wednesday!"

Mary apologized and helped me empty my bladder. As it turned out, that was the last time she was ever late. Her life soon became less hectic.

"That's great," said Molly.

I agreed, "Mary is a good attendant, and I need more women like her. Mary can help me during the day but can't get me up in the morning. In the meantime, my mom said she would help me get up while I tried to find someone."

"Hey," said Molly "I'll roll into the kitchen and make us some lunch."

"OK, I'll sit here and wait for the phone to ring." I got a few more calls that morning, but nothing panned out. Then Molly and I enjoyed a great lunch together. Molly stayed a while and then soon rolled out my door.

As you can see, good help is hard to find but the alternative is living in a nursing home. Nursing homes are fine for a lot of people, but not for me. Not yet. So, while it is difficult and time consuming to look for a good attendant, it is so worth it when you find one.

In the following chapter, I share my personal journey. Life has taught me many things and believe it or not, I wouldn't change *anything*. I appreciate everything that has happened thus far.

CHAPTER 9

THIS WASN'T WHAT I EXPECTED

I've been a woman on wheels since 1990. Am I happy about it? Not always. In fact, some days I'm so mad that I could explode. But, you can't live in what I call a "state of hate." It isn't healthy. I know people who are angry 24/7. They are always mad or upset about something. That seems like such a waste of energy to me! I've read that it takes fewer muscles to smile than it does to frown. I know life isn't easy. But when life gives you something unexpected, try to see it as an opportunity to learn something new and gain a different perspective.

I was 25 years old when I was a passenger in an SUV that rolled over, leaving me a quadriplegic and paralyzed from the chest down. I don't want you to feel pity but instead, compassion. Life is too darn short to sit around feeling sorry for yourself! Shortly after my accident, I was diagnosed with depression. I understand what it is, what causes it—and I control it using my personal motto: "Feel it, Think it, Write it, Say it!"

I never deny my feelings. If I'm happy, I laugh. If I'm sad, I cry. Then I think about my feelings and write in my journal. Some of my best poetry comes from my depression. Finally, I talk about my thoughts and feelings with my therapist, who I began seeing 3 years before my injury.

February 11, 1990, was a beautiful day. It was unseasonably warm, like early spring. The sky was blue, without a cloud in sight. It was the kind of day that made you feel like you should be outside enjoying it. There was no hint that this would be the day that would change my life forever.

I awoke at 7:30 a.m., as usual on a Sunday morning, and ate a bowl of cereal. The phone rang. It was Debbie and Sharon. The three of us, who rarely shared the same days off, found we had the day free and wanted to enjoy it together.

Debbie and Sharon suggested we all meet later that morning, so at about 10:00 a.m., we met in the apartment parking lot. We took off in Debbie's sport utility vehicle because it had the most gas. We had no real destination when we drove off. We thought about going to the St. Louis Zoo, but after a discussion, we decided to go to Hermann, Missouri, which was a drive of just under 2 hours.

Hermann is a small Missouri river town with antique dealers, wineries, and rolling hills with breathtaking views. Upon our arrival in the early afternoon, we got some lunch at a winery, and drove around through town enjoying the breezes blowing in our hair. At one of our stops along the way, we met three other women who told us about another cool place to visit, and we were on our way. I buckled my seat belt, and we were off with the sun shining as we gazed upon the beautiful surroundings. I didn't think life could have gotten any better! Good friends and good times.

While we were following the women we had just met, Debbie and I realized it was Sunday night and the new *Simpsons* cartoon would be on. We passed the ladies ahead of us to let them know we wouldn't be accompanying them on their journey.

As we headed back to St. Louis, we were riding down Highway 94, near Marthasville, Missouri. I was sitting in the front seat, and Sharon was in the back seat. I looked at Debbie and chuckled, "I wonder what Homer, Marge, Bart, Lisa, and Maggie are going to be up to this week?"

Sharon answered, "I don't know why you two like that Simpson cartoon. It's so stupid." Just then Sharon dropped her purse and the contents went everywhere.

Then Debbie and I said in unison, "D'oh!" and we laughed, knowing we'd done Homer Simpson proud.

That's the last thing I remember before I heard the sirens. The sirens. God were they loud. The sound filled my ears.

The next thing I knew, I was lying in a field of grass, questioning a paramedic who was kneeling beside me. "Why can't I move my arms or legs? Why can't I stand up?" I could hear the sound of a helicopter that was later to take me to Barnes Hospital in St. Louis. I don't remember the ride. It was surreal. I was there, I knew I was there, but it wasn't real. It felt like I was dreaming— a really bad dream at that! I never felt as if I was going to die. Death wasn't knocking on my door, but I knew something was different. Very different.

At the time of the accident, I was an average 25-year-old woman, trying to make my way in life with an optimistic attitude. I had no limiting factors in my life other than the average challenges of living on a small budget. Anyone who knows me will tell you I have always been a happy-go-lucky, fun-loving person with a purpose in life. My goals and ambitions were similar to others my age. My weakness? I guess my weakness would be wearing my emotions on my sleeve. My dramatic flare persuaded my 1983 high school senior class to declare me as "Most likely to win an Oscar," and my father often said to me, "Kathryn Claire Rodriguez, you are being overly dramatic!" That is why, to this day, I don't enjoy playing poker. If life is good or bad, I just can't hide it.

Four days prior to this accident, I had found the job of my dreams as a social director for two brand-new apartment communities. Good recreation jobs are hard to find, and I was waiting for an opportunity like this to use my degree in Recreation. Previously, my employment history in sales and marketing had consisted of experiences that never gave me what I wanted, but this new position consisted of running social programs, leading fitness classes, and meeting other recreational needs of the tenants. The compensation included a free apartment, full health benefits, and a monthly stipend. This was just what I was looking for, and I was ecstatic! I could finally do what I do best—organize fun.

The job would now have to be done by someone else.

I am so grateful for my family. My family was (and is) incredible. My father, Joseph Rodriguez (he didn't have a middle name, as he always said, "My family was too poor for middle names"), was raised in South St. Louis. His mother's uncle ran a cigar-making business, but it closed when Castro invaded Cuba, making Cuban tobacco unavailable. My grandfather, John Rodriguez, was a founder and first President of the Spanish American Society of St. Louis. My father's parents came to America from Spain in 1917 without much more than what they could carry. Dad was a great follower of the "Do It Yourself" philosophy that his parents had instilled in him.

My mother, Claire Rita Burke, was born in Ottawa, Ontario in Canada, and she grew up in New Jersey. She was the oldest of five siblings and went to school in New York to learn how to operate a key punch machine. (That was how they used to file records and information before computers.) She also worked for a phone company as a messenger. Soon after that, a friend introduced her to a Ricky Ricardo look-alike named Joe Rodriguez, and they married in 1945.

They lived with my father's parents in South St. Louis, where Spanish was spoken ninety percent of the time. My mother admits, "I couldn't understand a word, but the food was great!" My father was very proud of his Spanish heritage and was elated when my sister spent a year attending La Universidad Complutense de Madrid in Spain to become a Spanish teacher.

I am the sixth of seven children. Bob and Joe were born in the late 1940s. Pat, Dennis, and Eileen were children of the 1950s, and Tom and I came along in the mid 1960s. We are a somewhat close-knit family, considering that we never lived all together under the same roof at one time, which was to my parents' advantage. I was born the same year Bob left for college, on October 15, 1964, the day the St. Louis Cardinals won the World Series.

How my mom and dad managed to feed, clothe, and produce seven determined children is beyond me. I never remember ever going without. What was provided was what was needed, and anything beyond that was your own responsibility.

Right after the accident, Carroll, Pat's wife, was of great help to me. She had experience working in social services. She started to investigate programs and services that would help me live with my disability. Applying for disability benefits isn't an easy process. Because I had no health insurance at the time, Medicaid, the state insurance program for the poor, would cover my medical expenses and 6 months of hospitalization. I spent 2 months in the Intensive Care Unit at Barnes' Hospital and 4 months in the rehabilitation program at St. John's Mercy Medical Center. I can't thank these two institutions enough for their great nursing care and services. The real bummer today is that most people don't get the length of stay I did. We can thank insurance companies for this.

My brother Bob and sister-in-law Linda (Joe's wife) started the legal process against the manufacturer of the sport utility vehicle in which I was a passenger on that fateful day. The day after the accident, Bob and my dad and John Wallach, of the law firm Hoffman and Wallach, were at the scene of the accident.

Regarding the accident, some people have asked me if I am mad at Debbie who was driving the SUV that rolled over. I am not. Debbie came to see me a lot. I think it must have been hard for her, since she was the driver. But I knew that my family was taking legal recourse, and

Debbie had to be part of it. So I was going to let a jury weigh the issues and come to their own conclusions.

Little did I know at the time of my injury that it would take two separate 3-month-long trials, one in 1995 and one in 1997, and a 10-year legal battle, before my case would settle. I truly believe that what doesn't kill us makes us stronger.

As I lay in that hospital bed with my mind reeling, I learned that my sister Eileen relocated her family from Kansas City to St. Louis to help out. That was so nice of her to do so. She uprooted her husband, Bill, and her then 2-year-old daughter, Maddie. Eileen, who is 7 years my senior, grew up wiping my butt and braiding my hair. And here she was, ready to do it all over again.

My mother was the first person to learn how to catheterize me. As a can-do woman, she was ready and willing to take on this new challenge. She watched the nurse cath me and then the nurse watched my mom do the cath. Mom felt good about it and announced that there would be a family picnic at their house the next week.

My brother Tom came to the hospital and picked me up for my outing. I arrived at my parent's house and everyone was really excited. "Katie's here!" I heard my sister Eileen yell. Our family get-togethers can get quite hectic and full of activity. When it was time, my brothers put me on my parent's bed and Mom came in to cath me. Unfortunately, she couldn't put the tube where it needed to be. She forgot where to put it. Both of us were very frustrated. Sadly, I had to go back to St. John's Hospital to have my bladder emptied.

On the ride back to Mercy Medical Center, I again realized just how dependent I was going to be on others. I had no real control over my body anymore. I was pissed off—not only because I couldn't pee, but because this was only the beginning of the challenges that lay ahead of me. The nurses showed my mother the cathing process again, and she has had it down-pat since then.

After 6 months of hospitalization and rehabilitation, I moved back into my parent's home on August 10, 1990. However, before I was to be finally discharged from the hospital, my mother and I were to spend one night together in the model apartment on the rehab floor. Mom was going to be my primary caregiver. She had mastered the cath and could transfer me with assistance.

We went to sleep and awoke to a morning full of frustration. Everything went wrong! This was the first time Mom had to take care of my entire body from head to toe since I was a baby. Dressing a paralyzed body requires a lot of rolling, pushing, and tugging. I think it wore her out. She got me into my wheelchair, and I had a bowl of cereal. I put on some lipstick and barely made it down to rehab in time for my therapy session. The only thing that saved our sanity that morning was keeping our hopes high that things would improve. I again realized how difficult life was going to be. The rest of my life would be instructing individuals on how to care for me and my body, and I was exhausted after doing it for just 24 hours!

I had to learn how to live with two people I had not lived with under the same roof in 6 years! The home I grew up in was not at all accessible but fortunately, my parents had moved in 1986 to a modest four-bedroom split level home that turned out to have an adequate amount of accessibility. While the thought of living with my parents again seemed like something I didn't want to do, I was glad and thankful they were there for me when I needed them. Looking back on that experience, there was really more good than bad. My parents came through like champs.

A week out of rehab, my mom gave me the book *Joni* by Joni Erickson Tada. This is only one of many books by Joni. She's a quad, too. I sat in my parents' backyard, read the book, and cried and cried, and cried some more. It felt good knowing there was someone out there who knew what I was going through.

Mom, Dad, and I developed a routine after a while. Mom did my caths and dressed me. Then my parents grabbed me on either end and transferred me into my wheelchair.

Carroll researched social service agencies that offered respite care. Respite care gives people a break from each other. It can prevent burnout on both sides. Having a helping hand would give my folks a break, and give me a taste of independent living.

Early on, Carroll and Eileen were my afternoon attendants. They both learned how to cath me and transfer me in and out of their vehicles. Every other week, Carroll and I went on trips of investigation throughout the St. Louis area.

One day Carroll and I went to the Missouri Division of Vocational Rehabilitation (DVR) office, so that I could be assigned a counselor to help me look at my employment options. Carroll was transferring me from the car seat to my wheelchair, when my wheelchair started rolling away. We'd forgotten to secure the locks on my chair. We both started laughing. Carroll had my legs between her legs, my arms were wrapped around her shoulders, and she was about to drop me when a young man came by, grabbed the wheelchair, and held it still while Carroll put me in it. We thanked him and laughed some more.

A few months later, my sister Eileen took me to give my first "disability awareness" presentation. It was raining buckets that day as Eileen loaded me and my manual wheelchair into her car, but we made it. The high school students in attendance that day learned about living life with a disability, and they asked me some pretty interesting questions as well. Educating and motivating others has been therapeutic, and it has helped me face and endure my life as a quadriplegic. I had found my calling.

My next step toward independence occurred when La Petite Day Care donated a 1983 Ford van to my family. I guess it helped that my oldest brother Bob was President of the corporation at that time. I was ecstatic! Another set of wheels to help free me from my multiple limitations. Bob had the white day care van painted blue, giving her the name "Big Blue." The van was wonderful, but it needed adaptations for me to be a passenger.

It was back to DVR again. This is a state government program helping persons with disabilities to further their education or gain employment. Most states have this type of program or something similar to it. I learned that, because of my limited income, I was eligible to receive their assistance. DVR purchased a lift, lowered the floor, and installed insulation and tie downs (a set of belts that secure a wheelchair to the floor) in my van. This was great! No more transfers in and out of cars by my pit crew of assistants in inclement weather. I was good to go and ready to roll!

With my new vehicle, I was ready to hire a personal care attendant and experience even more independence. I put an ad in a community newspaper. I hired Kara, my first attendant, to work 3 days a week for a couple of hours each day. My parents covered the cost of paying my attendant $5.00 an hour.

Kara was married, had no children, and lived only 10 minutes away. She had a peaceful demeanor and was very patient. We were both in our late 20s, and we laughed at the same things. It was great to be out and about with her. Kara made me feel safe whether she was driving my van or helping me with my personal care. It was difficult exposing my body to a new person, but if I was going to be independent, I had to accept this part of being disabled. We went out for ice cream, to the library, and just had fun. With her I had 2 hours of total freedom, and it was liberating!

Having lived with my parents for 15 months, it became evident it was time for a change. My brother Tom and I had lived together before my auto accident, so we thought we'd give it a try once again. I had some reservations and was anxious, but overall I was primed for independent living.

Tom and I started combing the papers for homes to rent, and joined a house-locating service. We developed a list of what we needed; measurements, accessibility requirements, and rooms for Tom, an attendant, and me.

We called property owners and asked them if their homes were accessible. Many said "Yes," but when we went out to look, we were often disappointed. Their interpretation of accessibility was different from ours. Some property owners thought that one or two steps were no big deal, but one step is one too many for a person who uses a wheelchair.

After searching to the point of exhaustion, we finally found a 900-square-foot house that met our basic needs. It was a three-bedroom home with a walk-out basement. It was nearly perfect. The only adaptation needed before I could move in was a ramp over the two steps to the front door.

The next step was developing a budget. My income consisted of my Social Security check; a monthly contribution from my parents, my brothers, and sister; and food stamps. I received 3 hours of attendant care, five mornings a week from Medicaid, through the Missouri Division of Aging. Things were going to be tight, but I was used to that. Growing up in a large family means that there's not always enough to go around.

Tom moved his stuff in December 1991, and Pat built a beautiful wooden ramp from the driveway to the front door with an L-shaped turn. The rest of the house just had to be touched up and cleaned. Our simple home had a partially finished basement where Tom slept. The smallest bedroom on the first floor served as my office, and Tom built a desk for me by using a kitchen counter top resting on three wooden cabinets with doors. I could roll my wheelchair up to the desk and reach my speakerphone and other items. The bathroom was cramped, but workable. My shower chair straddled the bathtub.

I moved in on January 1, 1992. Kara assisted me in the transition, but she soon had to move on because she was expecting her first child. I put another ad in the paper, looking for a personal care attendant, and Mom said she would help whenever I needed her.

What really changed things for me was meeting Steven Banister in 1993 at the Missouri State Capitol in Jefferson City while advocating for funding to allow people with disabilities to live independently. I was there as a volunteer for Paraquad (a St. Louis Center for Independent Living), and my mission was to testify before the House Appropriations Committee in support of funding for the Personal Care Attendant program. Steve was there training consumers to be self-advocates.

At that time, Steve was the program manager for Services for Independent Living, the Columbia Center for Independent Living serving twenty mid-Missouri counties. After the testimony, our group visited with the governor's aide in the governor's office. As we were preparing to leave, I rolled over to Steve and asked him where he lived. He said, "In Columbia. Where do you live?"

I said, "St. Louis."

Steve said, "I grew up in St. Louis, and my parents live in Manchester."

"Cool. Next time you're in St. Louis, look me up," I said as we walked the corridors of the capital.

Being a strong advocate came naturally to both Steve and me. We were both passionate about lobbying our state legislators to better serve the needs of Missouri's citizens with disabilities. I guess my disability made me so ardent. Steve, who holds a degree in rehabilitation psychology, was just as committed.

Steve is so patient and caring. After a year and a half, he became my best friend. Soon after that, we were intimately dating so I figured that he had to learn how to do my catheterization. I asked my overnight attendant Lisa if she would feel comfortable showing Steve how to cath me. She said, "Sure. No big deal." The next night she came in, laid me down, removed my pants, and put my legs in the "frog-like" position, with the heels of my feet touching each other. Lisa then went into the living room and asked Steve to come and view the cath procedure.

Lisa cathed me and explained what she was doing while Steve looked on in a caring and loving way. Lisa removed the cath tube, and Steve said, "Is that it?"

Lisa responded with, "Yes, but always remember to keep everything as clean and sterile as possible."

Steve said, "OK, thanks Lisa," and walked out of the room.

Lisa and I looked at each other and I said, "Oh my God, this is the first man I have ever allowed to cath me."

Lisa said, "Really?"

"Yes," I continued. "I'm not sharing this body with just any man!" We both cracked up, and I then realized that Steve was "it." I had met my soul mate and it felt good. It felt like a warm fuzzy blanket on a cold winter's night.

Steve is the yin to my yang. He knows everything about me and hasn't run away yet! In 1999, he moved in with me at about the same time Tom found his wife Margie. It was cool how things worked out.

It was also at this time when my legal ordeal settled. This was great for so many reasons. First, I could pay back my family and do other nice things for them. Second, I could step off the state's dole and pay for things on my own. Finally, it meant that Steve and I could marry. If we had married before, I would have lost all my benefits and support systems. It seems to me that the systems that support us often limit us. There has got to be a better way, and I wish I had the answers. But I don't.

Together, Steve and I have worked out an efficient personal care assistance system. During the week, I have an aide in the morning and one at night. Steve does my afternoon and weekend care. Our afternoons are spent giving presentations to businesses and schools, attending meetings, writing, volunteering, and selling our Access-

Sacks and our children's book *Aunt Katie's Visit*. While this book targets children at an elementary-school level, kids of all ages and adults tell me how fun and educational it is. You can purchase our products on our website at www.access-4-all.com

I have always been into fitness and good health and my wheels have not stopped me. In 1995, I began using an electric "bike," The Ergys 2, a Functional Electrical Stimulation (FES) indoor stationary leg cycle. It has a big seat and a streamlined body that is connected to a box that houses the computer. I wear biking "shorts" with electrodes already sewn in them. In the morning, my attendant puts my bike shorts on, puts gel on each electrode so the stimulation won't burn my skin, and then she transfers me onto the bike. I try to ride two times a week, cycling 2 to 4 miles each time.

This cycle has helped me in many ways. First and foremost are the direct benefits to my legs and cardiovascular system. It has started to firm and tone the muscles in my legs. As a former aerobics instructor, you can imagine how happy I was to discover I could still exercise! While my cycling now takes over an hour, from start to finish, it's time well spent.

In 2005, I discovered the Enabling Mobility Center (EMC), a place to work out, whether you use a wheelchair, scooter, walker or cane. The environment is fun and supporting and the people who work at the EMC are physical and occupational therapists who want to empower their participants. There are arm cycles, weight lifting equipment, and other ways to exercise. The research and programs at the EMC are a collaboration between Washington University's Program in Occupational Therapy and Paraquad, our local center for independent living. Their EMC website is at http://enablemob.wustl.edu/

When I started lifting weights my combined total was 60 pounds. After a month, I increased it to 170 pounds. Again, that's not all together, but the total I lift exercising my biceps, pectoral, lateral and deltoid muscles. Also, after a month of going twice a week, I lost seven pounds, take less baclofin (medicine to control body spasms) and the usual pain in my left shoulder is gone.

Having a disability does not mean a person should give up on personal health but instead, you should keep yourself in shape to the best of your abilities. Obviously, if you weigh less, you are easier to care for in many ways and good health means few trips to the doctor.

There are those who think that, because I fully accept my life as a woman on wheels and I am financially able to take care of my body's many needs, that I have it easy. While I'm the happiest I've ever been in many ways, I sure do miss doing my own hair, dancing the way I used to, and wearing my 4-inch gray snakeskin pumps! God, I really loved those shoes. I really did. In fact, I miss all forty of my high-heels and other fun shoes. But high heels, paralyzed ankles, and foot peddles just don't work well together.

Life goes on and so have I. Yes, life's imperfections are frustrating and I wish bad things didn't happen. But challenges are opportunities to learn.

The Gift of Imperfection

I like things all neat in a row.
I like to hang on. I just won't let go.
Why are there messes that get in the way?
Why am I mad when YOU won't go MY way?

OK God. Where are you coming from?
Yes . . . Imperfections aren't any fun.
Why is there pain and why does it hurt?
Why do I wish that life had no dirt?
Why can't I walk and have all that I need?
I long for a life of simplicity.

I look at my family, neighbors, and friends.
Hoping some day that their troubles will end.
It's not fair. I'd kick my foot if I could.
So here I'm writing the words that I should.

Hey! Wait a minute . . . I'm fulfilling my quest.
I'm writing this poem like I've written the rest.
The life I experience I am sharing with you.
I've found the job that I must do.

All of my years on planet Earth
Imperfection abound. Every death. Every birth.
Our soul's given a gift. The gift to feel.
The trouble and pain make it all real.
So I wish for all good and none of the bad.
But sorrow show's me why I should be glad.

CHAPTER 10

FINAL THOUGHTS

I hope this manual on how to find and how to be a good personal care attendant has given you an understanding of both sides. The attendant care relationship can be tricky to balance, but once it's going well, the feeling is wonderful. It's like the arms of a watch in motion, tick, tick, ticking. The two sides mesh when both work in unison, together, as a team.

From the perspective of a person with disability, a caring and able individual aide is liberating. For an attendant, it can be a rewarding job. Anyone can be an aide. A personal care attendant takes the time to make a difference in someone else's life. The rewards are like ripples on a lake, spreading out, beyond themselves.

If you want to assist a person and don't know how, try using a sentence like:

"Hi. Do you need some help? I'm not sure how to help you, but if you tell me how to I really would like to."

Be prepared if you receive a momentary look of shock on the person with a disability's face. They are often used to getting ignored.

If you want to ask a person about their disability, there are nice ways and not-so-nice ways. A few years ago, a self-proclaimed healer came into my house to do some energy work. She entered in with a huff, plopped down on my couch, and asked, "So, what's wrong with you?" I couldn't help myself. I just had to repeat her question to her in a slow word by word pace, "What . . . is . . . *wrong* . . . with me?" She realized her condescending ways and didn't know what to say. She was never invited over again because she was a very cold and impersonal person.

So instead, try asking questions in an inquisitive yet caring way. Here are some examples:

- "What happened that caused you to use a wheelchair?"
- "I'm sure using a wheelchair wasn't something you expected."
- "How did it happen?"
- "How long have you used a wheelchair?"
- "When did you become a wheeler?"
- "It must be frustrating having a disability. How long has it been?"
- "Can I get you anything?"
- "Do you need any assistance?"
- "Just tell me what to do."

And then, please listen and help the person without having that "death-sentence look" on your face. Would you want someone looking at you with that "aww, isn't life just tragic" look? Leave the sorrow somewhere else. You can show your concern without a look of devastation.

Honestly, if you come from love, anything you say or do is going to be fine. Just do your best, and remember we all make mistakes. But often, if a person with a disability sees that you are trying, she will realize that and then anything is possible. But, if you shut down in any way, you'll probably run into a dead end. Communication has to take place on both sides.

Finally, I want you to realize that what you think creates your reality. This sounds simple and easy to do, but most of us don't comprehend how powerful our thoughts really are. If there is one movie that I would recommend the entire human race see, it would be "What the Bleep Do We Know?" This movie stars Marlee Matlin, an actress with a hearing impairment, who is pretty grumpy about her life and what's happened to her in the past. The movie is about the power of thought and how both science and religion recognize the power of the messages we send to and from our brain. It's a movie that will make you think! I hope you see it and come away with a feeling of self empowerment and responsibility for your own reality.

My reality is I'm a woman on wheels, and I wouldn't change anything that's happened as a result. My "chair" has brought on some wonderful lessons, especially about love. Love of myself and love of others.

And in closing . . . Don't be afraid to ask for help, and be there when someone needs it.

The Shade

You can't keep someone in the shade
They'll whither, choke, and die
How can they grow, how will the know
What it's like to try?
Protection by prejudice
Is not the way to teach.
Try compassion and understanding
Extend beyond your reach.
Cultivate your being
Don't put yourself above.
Shed beams of light, flee from fright
Because everyone needs love.

Appendix A
Duty Spreadsheet

	MON.	TUES.	WED.	THUR.	FRI.	SAT.	SUN.
7 a.m.							
8							
9							
10							
11							
12 Noon							
1							
2							
3							
4							
5							
6							
7							
8							
9							
10							
11 p.m							

Appendix B
The Telephone
Interview Sheet

TELL THE CALLER:

- Your general location
- Smoking preferences
- Your disability, duties, and shifts
- Pets and/or living arrangements
- Salary and method of payment

ASK THE CALLER:

Do you have reliable transportation? _____

Tell me about your experiences with disabilities:

_____

_____

Other work experiences?

_____

_____

Current schedule? _____

_____

Name? _____

Address? _____

Phone number? _____

Age? _____

Arrange for an interview:

Interview time and date: _____

- Please bring two (2) work and two (2) personal references with you.
- Please call if you need to cancel our meeting.

Appendix C The Application Form

Date: _____

Name (first, middle, last): _____

Address:_____

_____

_____

Phone (home, cell): _____

Social Security number: _____

Driver's license number (state issued): _____

Birth date (mm/dd/yyyy): _____

Schooling (Please include name of school, the city/state, the years you attended, your degree, and your graduation dates):

High school: _____

College: _____

Other: _____

Employment history:

Employer 1: _____

Phone #: (   )_____

Dates of employment, from _____ to _____

Position/title: _____

Supervisor's name: _____

Reason for leaving: _____

Employer 2: _____

Phone #: ( )_____

Dates of employment, from _____ *to* _____

Position/title: _____

Supervisor's name: _____

Reason for leaving: _____

Employer 3: _____

Phone #: ( )_____

Dates of employment, from _____ *to* _____

Position/title: _____

Supervisor's name: _____

Reason for leaving: _____

When are you available to work?

_____

What mornings/days/evenings are best? _____

Are you available on short notice? _____

Have you been convicted of a felony/misdemeanor/
other offense? _____

Please explain _____

_____

Are there any jobs that you would not want to do
(duties of the job description)? _____

If you have classes or other set commitments, please list
them.

Appendix D
Employment
Reference Form

Reference 1.

Name: _____

Phone # (   ) _____

Company: _____

Address/City/State: _____

_____

Relationship to you: _____

May I contact this person? _____

Reference 2.

Name: _____

Phone # (   ) _____

Company: _____

Address/City/State: _____

_____

Relationship to you: _____

May I contact this person? _____

Reference 3.

Name: _____

Phone # ( ) _____

Company: _____

Address/City/State: _____

_____

Relationship to you: _____

May I contact this person? _____

I declare that all information provided is true and complete. My signature on this document provides permission to contact my references for more information and conduct a criminal background check if necessary.

Signature: _____

Date: _____

Appendix E Police Background Check Authorization Form

Name: _____

Address: _____

_____

Phone number: ( ) _____

Date of birth: _____

Place of birth: _____

Social Security Number: _____

Driver's license number: _____

   State issued: _____

Race: _____

Sex: _____

Height: _____

Weight: _____

I hereby authorize the (location) _____ Police Dept. to release of police information regarding arrest and conviction information.

I attest that the above information is correct.

Signature:_____

Date: _____

Appendix F Disability-Related Resources

INTERNET SITES—STATE, LOCAL, AND NATIONAL RESOURCES

Many of the links below were given to me by the Special School District of St. Louis County. I appreciate their sharing this information.

Attendant Care Training

Access-4-All, Inc.
314-481-0633
www.access-4-all.com
Contact for training information.
Specialized disability organizations will train disability specific needs

United Cerebral Palsy
http://www.ucp.org

Epilepsy Foundation
www.epilepsyfoundation.org

National Multiple Sclerosis Society
www.nmss.org

Muscular Dystrophy Association
www.mdff.org

The Alzheimer's Association
800-272-3900
www.alz.org
Provides classes on attendant care for individuals with memory loss

Centers for Independent Living
For a list of all U.S. centers go to
www.ilru.org

Caregivers

National Family Caregivers Association
www.nfcacares.org

Wellspouse
www.wellspouse.org

The Caregivers Marketplace
www.caregiversmarketplace.com

Elder Care
www.ec-online.net

Disability/General Information

ADA Document Center
www.jan.wvu.edu/links/adalinks.htm

National Information Center for Children and Youth with Disabilities (NICHCY)
www.nichcy.org

National Organization on Disability
www.nod.org

National Rehabilitation Information Center (NARIC)
www.naric.com

Office of Special Education & Rehabilitative Services (OSERS)
www.ed.gov/about/offices/list/osers/index.html?src=mr

World Institute on Disability
www.wid.org

IDEA Practices Law & Regulations
www.ideapractices.org

PHYSICAL DISABILITY RESOURCES

Assistive Technology

Abledata
www.abledata.com

Alliance for Technology Access
www.ataccess.org

Assistive Tech
www.assistivetech.net

Rehabilitation Engineering & Assistive Technology Society of North America
www.resna.org

Cerebral Palsy

4 My Child
www.cerebralpalsy.org

National Institute of Neurological Disorders & Stroke: Cerebral Palsy
www.ninds.nih.gov/disorders/
cerebral_palsy/cerebral_palsy.htm

United Cerebral Palsy (UCP)
http://www.ucp.org

U.S. Cerebral Palsy Athletic Association
www.ndsaonline.org

Employment

Job Accommodation Network
www.jan.wvu.edu

Independent Living, Advocacy, Personal Assistance Services

Centers for Independent Living
www.ILRU.org

Multiple Sclerosis

Multiple Sclerosis Association of America
www.msaa.com

National Multiple Sclerosis Society
www.nmss.org

Muscular Dystrophy

Muscular Dystrophy Association
www.mdausa.org

Muscular Dystrophy Family Foundation
www.mdff.org

Spina Bifida

Spina Bifida Association of America
www.sbaa.org

Spinal Cord Injury

National Spinal Cord Injury Association
www.spinalcord.org

Paralyzed Veterans of America
www.pva.org

Worlds Wheelchair Culture
www.paralinks.net

SENSORY DISABILITY RESOURCES

Deaf, Hard of Hearing

Deaf Resource Library
www.deaflibrary.org

National Association for the Deaf
www.NAD.org

Vision Impairment

American Foundation for the Blind
www.afb.org

National Federation of the Blind
www.nfb.org

COGNITIVE DISABILITY RESOURCES

Attention Deficit Disorder (ADD)

Attention Deficit Disorder Association (ADDA)
www.add.org

Children & Adults with Attention
Deficit/Hyperactivity
www.chadd.org

Autism/Asperger Syndrome

Autism Society of America
www.autism-society.org

Judevine Center for Autism
www.judevine.org

Brain Diseases and Disorders/
Traumatic Brain Injury

Alzheimer's Association
www.alz.org

Brain Injury Association of America
www.biausa.org

Traumatic Brain Injury National Data Center
www.tbindc.org

Developmental Disabilities

Association for Retarded Citizens
www.thearc.org

National Down Syndrome Society
www.ndss.org

Epilepsy/Seizure Disorder

Epilepsy Foundation of America
www.epilepsyfoundation.org

Mental Health/Emotional Health

Bi-polar and Affective Brain Disorders
www.pendulum.org

National Alliance for the Mentally Ill
www.nami.org

Index

RELATED TITLES FROM DEMOS MEDICAL PUBLISHING:

Barrier-Free Travel: A Nuts and Bolts Guide for Wheelers and Slow Walkers, 2nd Edition, by Candy B. Harrington
ISBN 13: 9781932603095 $19.95

There Is Room at the Inn: Inns and B&Bs for Wheelers and Slow Walkers, by Candy B. Harrington
ISBN 13: 9781932603613 $21.95

Health Insurance Resources: A Guide for People with Chronic Disease and Disability, 2nd Edition, by Dorothy E. Northrop, MSW, ACSW; Stephen E. Cooper, and Kimberley Calder, MPS
ISBN 13: 9781932603347 $26.95

Insurance Solutions—Plan Well, Live Better: A Workbook for People with Chronic Illnesses or Disabilities, by Laura D. Cooper, Esq.
ISBN 13: 9781888799552 $24.95

The Disabled Woman's Guide to Pregnancy and Birth, by Judith Rogers, OTR
ISBN 13: 9781932603088 $24.95

To order these or any other Demos titles call toll-free, 1-800-532-8663, or visit us on the web at www.demosmedpub.com.

Demos

Demos Medical Publishing
386 Park Avenue South, Suite 301
New York, NY 10016